Mental Depression

About the Authors

Sibnath Deb is a senior faculty in Applied Psychology, Calcutta University, Kolkata. Earlier, he worked in a professional research company as Senior Research Manager and also in an international NGO as Research Officer. He is the Council Member of the International Society for Prevention of Child Abuse and Neglect (ISPCAN), USA; Founder Vice-President of the Indian National Society for Prevention of Child Abuse and Neglect; Founder Secretary of MIDSW—an NGO involved in child protection; and Member of the Board of Editors, Journal of Interpersonal Violence, USA. He was Steering Committee Member of the UN Secretary General Study on 'Violence Against Children'. He was also involved in ITPI Project as Country Project Leader which was launched in 12 countries under the sponsorship of OAK Foundation, Switzerland. Dr. Deb has to his credit many books including Children in Agony (recipient of *'Best Book Award 2007'*); Contemporary Social Problems in India; Styles of Parenting Adolescents: The Indian Scenario; Narcotic Drugs and Psychotropic Substances; Impact of Sexual Abuse and Child Abuse and Neglect: South Asian Scenario. Also, Dr. Deb has published more than 70 research papers and dealt with more than 40 large scale studies for different agencies like the WHO, IDRC, DFID, CRS, CARE, UNICEF, the Johns Hopkins University and so on. He can be reached at sibnath23@rediffmail.com/sibnath23@gmail.com

Anjana Bhattacharjee is a faculty in Psychology Dept., M.B.B. College, Agartala. Earlier, she worked in the Human Development and Research Institute, Kolkata as Project Director. She has six years research experience in the areas of mental depression, breast cancer, drug addiction, alcoholism and HIV/AIDS. She has published a number of papers in the national journals. Her areas of research interest include mental depression, drug addiction and problems of disadvantaged children.

Mental Depression

The Silent Killer

Sibnath Deb
M.Sc., LL.B., Ph.D.
and
Anjana Bhattacharjee
M.A., Ph.D.

CONCEPT PUBLISHING COMPANY, NEW DELHI-110 059

Cataloging in Publication Data—DK
Courtesy: D.K. Agencies (P) Ltd. <docinfo@dkagencies.com>

Deb, Sibnath, 1962-
Mental depression : the silent killer / Sibnath Deb and Anjana Bhattacharjee.
p. cm.
Study conducted at Kolkata, India.
Includes bibliographical references (p.
Includes index.
ISBN 13: 9788180695766
ISBN 10: 818069576X

1. Depression, Mental—India—Kolkata. 2. Depression, Mental—Treatment—India—Kolkata. 3. Mental health—India--Kolkata. I. Bhattacharjee, Anjana, joint author. II. Title.

DDC 362.250 954 14 22

ISBN-13: 978-81-8069-576-6
ISBN-10: 81-8069-576-X

First Published 2009

Published and Printed by
Ashok Kumar Mittal
Concept Publishing Company
A/15-16, Commercial Block, Mohan Garden
New Delhi (INDIA)

Phones : 25351460, 25351794
Fax : 091-11-25357109
Email : publishing@conceptpub.com

Foreword

The Book *"Mental Depression: The Silent Killer"* by Sibnath Deb, Ph.D. and Anjana Bhattacharjee, Ph.D is a key-work in the research and clinical intervention on patients suffering from depression in India. The suffering, the disease burden and the cost of unrecognized and sometimes discriminated forms of mental ill health of depression is a lamentable fact worldwide, despite the fact that extensive research has shown that depression is extremely widespread.

About 10.0-20.0% of populations in many countries have been found to be clinically depressed, needing medical, psychiatric and therapeutic help and medication. In Western Countries depression is part of the three most widespread, most costly and most important groups of illnesses in the triad of heart disease, cancer and depression. The tragic aspect of the neglect and stigmatisation of depression lies in the fact that like malnutrition and the ill health following from it, depression is often extremely well treatable through both psychological interventions and medication, alleviating a huge degree of suffering, lightening the burden of disease and saving huge amounts of costs to society which are created when depression is not treated. In addition, it is important to note that depression effects people of all ages from childhood through young adulthood into old age. Equally it needs to be diagnosed and treated in all ages and both in women and in men although it is more prevalent in women.

Sibnath Deb and Anjana Bhattacharjee's work has investigated depression as important mental illness. Today we know increasingly more of the disease chemistry and structure in the brain. Their book is an important contribution to the research and treatment of depression worldwide and must be read and taken note of, not only by psychiatrists but by all medical professionals in general medicine, internal medicine and other medical fields as well as in psychology and by professionals concerned with the physical health and social well being of clients from childhood into all age. The authors provide an invaluable guide to diagnosis of depression, provides tools to assist the illness and suggests valuable ways for treatment. In this authors do not only concentrate on the medical and mental health aspect but also on the important need for the inclusion of the family, the social network and the community. A multi modal approach of mental health treatment including psychological treatment and medication as well as the involvement of the social network, the family and the community creates an overall integrated ecologically approach to the illness of depression through which Sibnath Deb and Anjana Bhattacharjee propose a most effective and efficient way to treat this much under-diagnosed and marginalised but extremely common and well to treat illness.

This book *"Mental Depression: The Silent Killer"* will help to dissimilate in India the knowledge about the nature, the symptoms, the consequences and the treatment of depression. The book will also certainly help to raise awareness and provide tools for effective intervention and treatment of the illness. Therefore, this book must not be missed by any doctor practicing in the field, not only of psychiatry but from child and adolescent mental health to general medicine and other medical specialties as well as all professionals working in the field of general physical health, community health and social well-being in India. The book is a most informative and valuable read for all professionals concerned.

Prof. Tilman Fürniss

M.D., P. Phil., FRC Psych (London)
Professor of Child and Adolescent Psychiatry,
Adult Psychiatrist
University Hospital, University of Muenster, Germany

Preface and Acknowledgements

Depression is known as silent disease since it slowly affects an individual and the individual remains totally unaware at the initial stage. Most of the people get depressed from time to time for various reasons. In the 21st century with the advancement of science and technology, life has become very much complicated and people suffer from stress and strain. Some people can cope with the situation while some can't. Expectation of common people is also going up day by day and in this regard media is playing a very significant role. When peoples needs and expectations are not fulfilled they eventually fall prey to depression. Latest statistics say that West Bengal is one of the states where a large number of people commit suicide every year because of severe mental depression. Another indication of increasing number of depressive patients is reporting of the same category of patients in the city mental health centres.

Given the above situation, the necessity of carrying out the systematic study on depression was reinforced with a view to understanding the socio-economic and demographic background of the depressive patients, their personality dispositions, self-esteem, emotional control, and suicidal tendencies. Further an effort was made to understand the perceived problems of the family members in dealing with depressive patients. Finally, the study proposed some need-based measures for family members for better care and management of depressive patients.

While carrying the study we have received full cooperation and support from the Faculty Members of the Department of Applied Psychology, Calcutta University. We are grateful to all of them.

The success of any research and/or fieldwork depends upon cooperation from different organizations for contacting the subjects of the study. We have received good cooperation from a number of Psychiatrists who helped us in collecting data. We are grateful to Dr. Satrajit Dasgupta, President of 'Antara'—A Mental Health Centre and Senior Psychiatrist, Dr. Japasish Chakraborty, Senior Resident Psychiatrist of 'A Centre for Human Mind', Jadavpur, Kolkata, Dr. D. Das, Psychiatrist, R.G. Kar Medical College, Kolkata and Dr. D. Chowdhury, Psychiatrist—a private practitioner. Our acknowledgement is due to all of them.

For comparison of data of depressive patients, we covered an equal number of normal population matched in terms of age and gender. We are thankful to all the depressive patients, their family members and normal population for their wholehearted cooperation in providing necessary information from time to time for the interest of the study.

We are indebted to the Librarian of the Department of Applied Psychology, University of Calcutta and other staff members for their assistance. Gratitude is extended to authors of all the books, articles and research papers that have added academic value to my work.

We are also grateful to Prof. Tilman Furniss, M.D., M.Phil, ERCPsych, Dept. of Child and Adolescent Psychiatry, University Hospital Muerster and Prof. Sudha Bhogle, Ph.D., Dept. of Psychology, Bangalore University for reviewing the document and giving their valuable feedback.

Finally, we express out heartfelt gratitude to all our family members for their continuous support and help.

Every effort has been made to produce an error-free document. However, if there is any error or mistake the same is regretted. Any further suggestion on the work will be highly appreciated.

Sibnath Deb
M.Sc., LL.B., Ph.D.
Anjana Bhattacharjee
M.A., Ph.D.
Department of Applied Psychology
University College of Science and Technology,
Calcutta University
92, A.P.C. Road, Kolkata-700009, India

Contents

List of Tables

List of Figures

1

Introduction

Depression: A Silent Killer

Depression, the silent killer has become one of the alarming crises in today's fast paced society. Even without the presence of any actual illness, major depression robs off all self worth, self-esteem, self-confidence and self-image. We live in a fast paced world. The pressures we are under to perform and produce results are insurmountable. And then there are the actions of those around us that sicken us to our souls and make us think that the world is a sad place to live in. There are days when we don't want to get out of bed. There are nights when we can't sleep. There are times when we wonder what exactly is the meaning and purpose of this life on earth and would anyone truly miss us if we were no longer around.

Depression is still looked upon as a taboo subject, which is ridiculous when we realize how many people suffer from depression. There are varying degrees of depression. Some mild, some quite severe and debilitating. The most severe of all is the degree of depression, which leaves the sufferer feeling alone, lost, and without hope for long periods of time culminating in suicide...the only way out the sufferer can see.

What does depression originate from? In this 21st century we are very much familiar with the term 'Mood'. Every normal individual experience a wide range of mood variations during their lifetime. Mood may be normal, elevated or depressed. When an individual experiences elevated mood, he shows expansiveness, flight of ideas, high self-esteem and grandiose ideas. On the contrary, an individual with depressed mood expresses lack of energy, low self-esteem, loss of interest and thoughts of death.

Major depressive disorder, commonly referred to as 'depression,' can severely disrupt one's life, affecting appetite, sleep, work, and relationships.

Mood disorder involves severe alterations in mood for prolonged period of time. The signs and symptoms of mood disorder include changes in activity level, cognitive abilities, speech and vegetative functions e.g.—sleep, appetite, sexual activity etc.

For mood disorder 'depression' is the most deadly one affecting a large number of population across the world. Depressive disorder occurs with alarming frequency at least 10 to 20 times more frequently than Schizophrenia. The lifetime prevalence rate of depression for males and females are 13% and 21% respectively (Kessler et al., 1994).

Depression is an emotional state of dejection, feeling of worthlessness, guilt accompanied by apprehension. Depression can be of two types—Endogenous and Exogenous. Endogenous depression is self-made, largely of ones own making without any apparent reason e.g.—observing colleague's prosper. Endogenous or reactive depression is due to factors beyond ones control such as noise, environment and so on.

In contrast to the normal emotional experiences of sadness, loss or passing mood states, clinical depression is persistent and can interfere significantly with an individual's ability to function. 'Depression' is a universal, timeless and ageless human affliction. It affects the way a person eats and sleeps, the way one feels about oneself, and the way one thinks about things. A depressive disorder is not the same as a passing blue mood. It is not a sign of personal weakness not a condition that can be willed or wished away. The economic cost of this disorder is high, but the cost in human suffering cannot be estimated.

Depression is rightly termed as the silent disease because it slowly affects an individual and the individual does not realise at the initial stage. Most of the people get depressed from time to time. With the advancement of the society in science and technology, life has become more complicated and we have to face competition everywhere. When people cannot cope with the stressful situation, when peoples' needs are not fulfilled, they eventually fall prey to depression.

Earlier, depression was considered as a disorder of middle aged or older people. Gradually this conception has changed. Nowadays it is evident that the most common age for onset of depression is youth or early adulthood (Burke et al., 1990). Klerman and Weissman (1989) were among the first to note that rates of depressive disorder were relatively higher in those born more recently. Another study carried out in the United States confirms the said findings (Burke et al., 1990 and 1991; Ryan et al., 1992; Lewinsohn et al., 1993).

Women experience depression about twice as often as men (Sorenson et al., 1991; Blazer et al., 1994). Many hormonal factors may contribute to the increased rate of depression in women—particularly such factors as changes in menstrual cycle, pregnancy, miscarriage, postpartum period, pre-menopause and post-menopause. Although men are less likely to suffer from depression than women, three to four million men in the United States are affected by the illness. Men are, however, less likely to admit depression.

The rate of suicide in men is four times that of women, though more women attempt it. Men's depression is often masked by alcohol or drugs, or by the socially acceptable habit of working excessively long hours. Depression typically shows up in men not as feeling of hopeless and helpless, but as being irritable, angry, and discouraged; hence depression may be difficult to recognize among men.

In Indian psyche, the 'male' identify tends to overshadow the limitations caused by any kind of mental problem. The position of women however differs. The marital status of a woman often acts as a determining factor of her position in her family as well as in the society. A girl's life is perceived as incomplete in Indian culture if she remains a spinster all her life. Even after marriage also, motherhood plays an important role in determining the social status of an woman. Such women are perceived as social burden and hence are more vulnerable to depression.

The concept and scenario of mental problem is changing very rapidly, yet in our country most of the people are not aware of mental illness. Here any mental problem is termed as 'Madness', Lack of awareness and stereotyped thoughts pushes us into the deep well of darkness. So, we often cannot understand their problems, their feelings and their unspoken pain. This negligence makes the depressed persons more sad and unhappy and hence prolongs their recovery.

The significance of Public health has been known for nearly 2,500 years and mood disorders continue to command major public health interest. The term 'mood disorders' group together a number of clinical conditions whose common and essential features are disturbance of mood, accompanied by related cognitive, psychomotor, psychophysiological and interpersonal difficulties.

Mood disorders are best considered as syndromes (rather than discrete diseases) that consist of a cluster of signs and symptoms that are sustained over a period of weeks to months, represent a marked departure from a persons habitual functioning and tend to recur often in periodic or cyclic fashion.

Diagnostic and Statistical Manual (DSM-IV) classifies mood disorders as Depressive Disorders (unipolar depression), the Bipolar Disorders, mood disorders due to a general medical condition and substance abused mood disorder (the last two are based on etiology). Depression is the most common mood disorder.

Depression is one of the major health problems affecting a large number of population especially younger generations across the world. It is estimated that in the next two/three years this disease will affect majority of the population.

The term 'depression' is used in everyday language to describe a range of experiences from a slightly noticeable and temporary mood decrease to a profoundly impaired and even life-threatening disorder. When used to describe a mood, the term conveys a temporary state of dysphoria that may last a few moments, hours or even a few days. As such, it is usually a normal reaction to an upsetting event, or even an exaggerated description of a typical event. Basically depression refers to a constellation of experiences including not only mood but also physical, mental and behavioural experiences that define more prolonged impairing and severe conditions that may be clinically diagnosable as the syndrome of depression.

Symptoms of Depression

Depressed people may differ from one another by the number, unique patterns and severity of the symptoms. The various symptoms of depression are:

Affective Symptoms

Depression is one of the several disorders generally called affective disorders, referring to the manifestations of abnormal affect or mood as a defining feature. The various affective symptoms of depression are:

(i) **Depressed Mood:** It is always present in a mild or severe form. In its mildest form, the individual experiences a flattering of affect, and as the depression increases, the individual is more miserable and unhappy. He becomes preoccupied with gloomy thoughts and tends to look on the dark side of the things. Thus, depressed mood, sadness, feeling low, down in the dumps or empty is typical. The depressed mood can be inferred from the person's facial expression and demeanor.

(ii) **Irritability:** Depressed individuals often exhibit irritability, e.g. persistent anger, a tendency to respond to events with angry outbursts or blaming others, or an exaggerated sense of frustration over minor matters. In children and adolescents, an irritable or cranky mood may develop a sad or dejected mood.

(iii) **Loss of Interest:** The experience of loss of interest or pleasure is one of the most common features of the depressive syndrome, according to many studies on depressed adults and teenagers of many different countries (Klinger, 1993). Depressed individuals often exhibit feeling loss of interest or pleasure, a feeling of "blah", listlessness and apathy. Nothing seems enjoyable—not even experiences that previously elicited positive feeling, including work and recreation, social interaction, sexual activity and the like. Pass times are no longer enjoyable; even pleasurable relationships with one's family and friends may no longer hold appeal or even become negative, and the individual may find it hard to think of things to do that might help to relieve the depression even temporarily.

Nothing can permanently raise his interest, nothing gives him pleasure, even when the person is accomplishing an important task, and there is little sense of satisfaction. Some severely depressed individuals often describe the loss of pleasure as seeing the world in black, white and gray with no colour.

Cognitive Symptoms

Some researchers have defined depression as a disorder of 'thinking', as some have defined it as a disorder of 'mood'. The important cognitive symptoms are:

(i) **Negativistic Thinking:** Depressed people typically have negative thoughts about themselves, their world and their future. The negativistic thinking is commonly irrational and distorted and represents very different interpretations of the self and the world during the depressed state than an individual would typically display when not depressed. This cognitive feature of depression has been given particular emphasis by some investigators, who note that thinking in such grim and self-critical ways actually makes people more depressed and prolong their depression.

(ii) **Guilt Feeling:** The depressed individuals often experience themselves as incompetent and worthless, and are relentlessly critical of their own act and characteristics. They often feel guilty as they dwell on their perceived shortcomings. The guilt feeling in depression varies from culture to culture, and it often does not appear in patients from African and Asian cultures, whereas in Europe, and U.S.A., about three in four patients exhibit guilt to some degree.

(iii) **Low Self-esteem:** It is a common attribute of depression. Individual may feel helpless to manage their lives and resolve problems. They may view their lives and futures as black and unrewarding with a persistent feeling that change is not only pointless but also essentially unattainable.

(iv) **Suicidal Thoughts:** Depressed individuals often think that they are superfluous in the world and they do not have any right to retain their lives any longer. Cognition reflecting hopelessness about one's ability to control desired outcomes may be common, and the resulting despair may also give rise to thoughts of wanting to die or to take one's own life. The suicidal thoughts range from a belief that others would be better off if the person was dead, to transient but recurrent thoughts of committing suicide, to actually specify plans of how to commit suicide. The frequency, intensity and lethality of these thoughts can be quite variable. Less severely suicidal individuals may report transient (1 to 2 minute), recurrent (once or twice week) thoughts. More severely suicidal individuals may have acquired materials (e.g. a rope or a gun) to be used in the suicide attempt and may have established a location and time when they will be isolated from others so that they can accomplish the suicide. Motivations for suicide may include a desire to give up in the face of perceived insurmountable obstacles or an intense wish to end an excruciatingly painful emotional state that is perceived by the person to be without end.

(v) **Impaired Mental Process:** In addition to negativistic thinking, depression is often marked by difficulties in mental processes involving concentration, decision-making and memory. The depressed person may find it enormously difficult to make even simple decisions, and significant decisions may seem beyond one's capacity altogether. Depressed patients often report problems in concentrating, especially when reading or watching television, and memory may be impaired (Watts, 1993). Memory problems, in fact, often lead depressed people to worry further that their minds are failing, and hence the problem becomes more dangerous.

Behavioural Symptoms

The important behavioural symptoms of depression are:

(i) **Social Withdrawal**: Depression leads to social withdrawal. Because of the apathy, diminished motivation and interest. It is common for depressed individuals to withdraw from social activities or reduce their typical behaviour. In severe depression, the individual might stay in the bed for prolonged periods.

(ii) **Psychomotor Changes**: Actual changes in movements, called psychomotor changes are often observed taking the form of being slowed down or agitated and restless. Some depressed individuals may talk and move very slowly, their faces show little animation with their mouths and eyes seeming to droop as if weighted down. Their speech is marked by pauses, fewer words, a monotonous voice and less eye contact (Cloitre et al., 1993). In severe forms, the depressed individual's activity is diminished, the voice fades and speech becomes an indistinct mumble and finally ceases, leading to mutism.

Somatic Symptoms

Some somatic symptoms are characteristic of depression and may even come to dominate the clinical picture. The various somatic symptoms are:

(i) **Reduced Energy:** It is a very frequent complaint (occurring in 93.0% of depressed patients as reported in a study by Buchwald and Rudick-Davis, 1993). Depressed patients feel a general loss of energy, quickly become tired and completely exhausted, and have vague feeling aches in the muscles and complain of headache. Depressed patients complain of listlessness, lethargy, feeling heavy and leaden, and lacking the physical stamina to undertake or complete tasks.

(ii) **Gastro-intestinal Symptoms:** The Gastro-intestinal symptoms are very common among depressed individuals like decrease in appetite, loss of interest in food, dryness of mouth and constipation and this decreased appetite results in weight loss. To some depressed individuals appetite changes may take the form of increased appetite with corresponding weight gain.

(iii) **Insomnia/Hypersomnia:** Sleep changes are one of the hallmarks of depression, and can take several forms like difficulty falling asleep, staying asleep or too much sleep. Depressed patients often experience what is called "Early Morning Awakening", which occurs 2-3 hours before the patient's usual time of waking up; usually with difficulty falling back asleep as a result he lies awake feeling un-refreshed and often restless and agitated. The patient thinks about the past failures and a gloomy future. It is this combination of 'early morning awakens' with 'depressive thinking' that is important in diagnosis. In some depressed patients, hypersomnia instead of early morning awakening may occur, yet they still report that the sleep was not refreshing.

(iv) **Loss of Libido:** Another important somatic symptom of depression is the loss of libido. Loss of libido occurs early in the development of depressive illness. Depressed men may complain of difficulty with erections, of an inability to ejaculate and finally of complete impotence. Among depressed women, amenorrhea and loss of sexual interest is common.

Besides, sometime depressive patients complain about palpitations, breathlessness, and pain in the chest, feeling dizzy, fainting, trembling, choking and sweating with a sense of impending doom.

Types of Depression

According to the Diagnostic and Statistical Manual of Mental Disorder (DSM-IV), Depressive disorder basically takes one of the three following forms:

- Major Depressive Disorder
- Dysthymic Disorder

Depressive Disorder not otherwise specified (including several forms of briefer on milder period of depression). These conditions are briefly described.

Major Depressive Disorder

(i) Essential Features: The essential features of major depressive disorder are a clinical course that is characterized by one or more major depressive episodes without a history of Manic, Mixed or Hypomanic episodes. The essential feature of a major depressive episode is a period of at least two weeks during which there is either depressed mood or the loss of interest or pleasure in nearly all activities. And the mood in a major depressive episode is often described by the depressed person as depressed, sad, hopeless, discouraged or 'down in the dumps'. Loss of interest or pleasure is nearly always present, at least to some degree. Individuals may report feeling less interested in hobbies, "not caring any more", or not feeling any enjoyment in activities that were previously considered pleasurable including sex. Besides these, other symptoms of major depressive disorder are:

- Feeling of hopelessness, pessimism.
- Feeling of guilt, worthlessness, helplessness.
- Decreased energy, fatigue, being "slowed down".
- Difficulty in concentrating, remembering and making decisions.
- Insomnia or hypersomnia.

- Loss of appetite and/or weight loss or over eating and/ or weight gain.
- Thoughts of death or suicide, suicidal attempts.

Other associative features of major depressive disorders are irritability, brooding, obsessive rumination, anxiety, phobias, excessive worrying over physical health, and complaints of pain (e.g. headaches or joint, abdominal or other pains). In children, separation anxiety may occur.

Major Depressive Disorder is often associated with high mortality. About 15.0% individuals with severe major depressive disorder die by committing suicide. Epidemiological evidence also suggests that there is a fourfold increase in death rates in individuals with Major Depressive Disorder who are over 55 years of age. Individuals with Major Depressive Disorder admitted to nursing homes may have a markedly increased likelihood of death in the first year.

Major Depressive Disorder may be preceded by Dysthymic Disorder (10.0% in epidemiological samples and 15.0-25.0% in clinical samples). It is also estimated that each year approximately 10.0% of individuals with Dysthymic Disorder alone have their first major depressive episode. Other mental disorders frequently co-occur with Major Depressive Disorder e.g. Substance—Related Disorders, Panic Disorder, Obsessive-Compulsive Disorder, Anorexia Nervosa, Bulimia Nervosa, Borderline Personality Disorder.

Major Depressive Disorder may be associated with chronic general medical conditions. About 20.0–25.0% of the individuals with certain medical condition (e.g.—diabetes, myocardial infarction, carcinomas, stroke etc.) may develop Major Depressive Disorder during the course of the general medical condition (*Source*: Diagnostic and Statistical Manual of Mental Disorder, IV).

(ii) Specific Culture, Age and Gender Features: Culture has a predominent influence on the experience and communication of symptoms of Major Depressive Disorder. In some cultures, Major Depressive Disorder may be experienced largely in somatic forms, rather than with sadness or guilt. Complaints of "nerves" and headaches (in Latino and

Mediterranean culture), of weakness tiredness or 'indolence' (in Chinese and Asian cultures), of problems of "heart" (in middle eastern cultures) or of being 'heartbroken' (among Hopi) may express the depressive experience. Major depressive disorder (Single or Recurrent) is twice as common in adolescents and adult females as in adolescents and adult males. Pre-pubertal children, boys and girls are equally affected. Certain symptoms such as Somatic Complaints, motor retardation, hypersomnia and delusions are less common in puberty than in adolescence and adulthood. Rates in men and women are highest in the 25-44 years age group, where as rates are lower for both men and women over age 65 years (*Source*: Diagnostic and Statistical Manual of Mental Disorder, IV).

Major Depressive Disorder may begin at any age, with an average age at onset being the mid 20's.

(iii) Prevalence: Studies of Major Depressive Disorder have reported a wide range of values for the proportion of the adult population with the disorder. The lifetime risk for Major Depressive Disorder in community samples has varied from 10.0 to 25.0% for men. The point prevalence of Major Depressive Disorder in adults in community samples has varied 2.0-3.0% for men (*Source*: Diagnostic and Statistical Manual of Mental Disorder, IV, p. 341).

Major Depressive Disorder is 1.5-3 times more common among first-degree biological relatives of persons with this disorder than among the general population. There is evidence for an increased risk of Alcohol Dependence in adult first-degree biological relatives, and there may be an increased incidence of Attention-Deficit/Hyperactivity Disorder in the children of adults with this disorder (*Source*: Diagnostic and Statistical Manual of Mental Disorder, IV, p. 341).

Dysthymic Disorder

(i) Essential Features: The essential feature of Dysthymic Disorder is a chronically depressed mood that occurs for most of the days for at least 2 years. Individuals with Dysthymic Disorder describe their mood as sad or "down in the dumps". In children, the mood may be irritable rather than depressed, and the required minimum duration is only 1 year.

Several studies suggest that the most commonly encountered symptoms of Dysthymic Disorder are:

- Feelings of inadequacy.
- General loss of interest or pleasure.
- Social withdrawal.
- Feeling of guilt or brooding about the past.
- Subjective feelings of irritability or excessive anger.
- Decreased activity, effectiveness or productivity.

In individuals with Dysthymic Disorder, vegetative symptoms (e.g. sleep, appetite, weight change, and psychomotor symptoms) appear to be less common than for persons in a Major Depressive Episode. When Dysthymic Disorder without prior Major Depressive Disorder is present, it is a risk factor for developing Major Depressive Disorder (10.0% of individuals with Dysthymic Disorder will develop Major Depressive Disorder over the next year). Dysthymic Disorder may be associated with Borderline, Histrionic, Narcissistic, Avoidant, and Dependent Personality Disorders. However, the assessment of features of a Personality Disorder is difficult in such individuals because chronic mood symptoms may contribute to interpersonal problems or be associated with distorted self-perception. Other chronic Axis I disorders are e.g., Substance Dependence or chronic psycho-social stressors may be associated with Dysthymic Disorder in adults. In children, Dysthymic Disorder may be associated with Attention-Deficit/Hyperactivity Disorder, Conduct Disorder, Anxiety Disorders, Learning Disorders, and Mental Retardation.

(ii) Associated Laboratory Findings: About 25.0-50.0% of adults with Dysthymic Disorder have some of the same polysomnographic features that are found in some individuals with Major Depressive Disorder e.g. reduced rapid eye movement, latency, increased REM density, reduced slow-wave sleep, impaired sleep continuity. Those individuals with polysomnographic abnormalities more often have a positive family history for Major Depressive Disorder (and may respond better to anti-depressant medications) than those with Dysthymic Disorder without such findings. Whether polysomnographic abnormalities are also found in those with "pure" Dysthymic Disorder (i.e., those with no prior history of Major Depressive Episodes) is not clear. Dexamethasone non-suppression in Dysthymic Disorder is not common, unless criteria is also met for a Major Depressive Episode.

(iii) Specific Age and Gender Features: In children, Dysthymic Disorder seems to occur equally in both sexes and often result in impaired school performance and social interaction. Children and adolescents with Dysthymic Disorder are usually irritable and cranky as well as depressed. They have low self-esteem and poor skills and are pessimistic. Among adults, women are two to three times more likely to develop Dysthymic Disorder than men.

(iv) Prevalence: The lifetime prevalence of Dysthymic Disorder (with or without superimposed Major Depressive Disorder) is approximately 6.0%. The point prevalence of Dysthymic Disorder is approximately 3.0%.

(v) Familial Pattern: Dysthymic Disorder is more common among first-degree biological relatives of people with Major Depressive Disorder than among the general population.

Depressive Disorder Not Otherwise Specified

The 'Depressive Disorder Not Otherwise Specified' category includes disorders with depressive features that do not meet the criteria for Major Depressive Disorder, Dysthymic Disorder, Adjustment Disorder with Depressed Mood, or Adjustment Disorder with Mixed Anxiety and Depressed Mood. Sometimes depressive symptoms can present as part of an Anxiety Disorder Not Otherwise Specified. Examples of Depressive Disorder Not Otherwise Specified include:

(i) **Premenstrual Dysphoric Disorder:** It occurs in most menstrual cycles during the past year, symptoms (e.g., markedly depressed mood, marked anxiety, marked affective liability, decreased interest in activities) regularly occurred during the last week of the luteal phase (and remitted within a few days of the onset of menses). These symptoms must be severe enough to markedly interfere with work, school, or usual activities and be entirely absent for at least 1-week post menses.

(ii) **Minor Depressive Disorder:** Episodes of at least 2 weeks of depressive symptoms but with fewer than the five items required for Major Depressive Disorder.

(iii) **Recurrent Brief Depressive Disorder:** It refers to depressive episodes lasting from 2 days up to 2 weeks, occurring at least once a month for 12 months (not associated with the menstrual cycle).

(iv) **Post Psychotic Depressive Disorder of Schizophrenia:** A major Depressive Episode that occurs during the residual phase of Schizophrenia.

(v) **A Major Depressive Episode** superimposed on Delusional Disorder, Psychotic Disorder Not Otherwise Specified, or the active phase of Schizophrenia.

(vi) Situations in which the clinician has concluded that a depressive disorder is present but is unable to determine whether it is primary, due to a general medical condition, or substance induced.

Sub-Types of Depression

In addition to the more formal diagnostic sub-types of depression currently included in the DSM-IV and ICD-IO, that are defined by severity or duration, there is an enormous need to consider the possible qualitative distinctions in depressions. As indicated by the heterogeneity of expressions of the features of depression, some seem more "biological" in presentation while others are more "psychological". Also, the depressions may vary considerably in their possible etiological factors, including both biological and psychological origins.

Historically, research has focused on the neuro psychotic, reactive-endogenous, and endogenous-non-endogenous sub-types, but the terms *psychotic* and *endogenous* have variously referred to severity or qualitative distinctions, or to absence of precipitating stressors, often with different investigators using the same term with different operational criteria. A theme cutting across the search for subtypes has been the idea that there are "biological" (endogenous) depressions that are diseases arising in the absence of environmental precipitants vs. 'psychological' depressions that stem from personality or situational factors. As Zimmerman et al., (1987) noted labels for "endogenous" depression have included vital severe, major incapacitating, psychotic, primary, retarded, melancholic, autonomous, and endogenomorphic, while "non-endogenous" depressions, have been variously termed neurotic, reactive, characterologic, atypical, secondary, mild, psychogenic, situational, and non-melancholic.

The following are clinically derived sub-groups based on descriptive features:

(i) **Melancholic Features:** It include loss of pleasure in all or almost all activities, lack of reactivity to pleasurable stimuli such that even good events, funny stories, or enjoyable experiences do not elicit any (or only a small amount) of positive reaction. Also, depression is regularly worse in the morning than evening (diurnal variation), the person shows excessive or inappropriate guilt, early morning awakening, marked psychomotor change (retarded or agitated), significant loss of appetite and weight loss. The person with melancholia may also experience the depression as having a distinct quality that is different from the kind of sadness felt after the death of a loved one. The melancholic sub-type of depression appears to predict a favourable response to anti-depressant medications (Jouce and Paykel, 1989; Rush and Weissenburger, 1994), and therefore might have important treatment implications. It has also been found to correlate with certain abnormal biological functions that some have speculated are indicators of an underlying depressive 'disease' (Rush and Weissenburger, 1994). Individuals who display the melancholic sub-type tend to show similar features during subsequent episodes (Coryell et al., 1994).

(ii) **Seasonal Pattern Depressions**: Seasonal pattern depressions refer to those that have an apparent regular onset during certain times of the year, and which also disappear at a characteristic time of the year. In the

Northern hemisphere, the most common pattern is autumn or winter depressions, clearing up in the spring, although some individuals experience regular summer depressions. The seasonal pattern has been observed in 15.0% of patients with recurrent mood disorders, including both unipolar and bipolar forms (Faedda et al., 1993). Qualitatively, such depressive episodes are especially marked by low energy, more sleeping, over-eating and weight gain, and craving for carbohydrate foods (Jacobsen et al., 1986).

(iii) **Depression With Psychotic Features:** Depression with psychotic features is usually a severe depression in terms of the general symptoms, and includes presence of either hallucinations or delusions. Typically, such hallucinations or delusions have a depressive theme, such as guilt due to the belief that one has caused a terrible misfortune, belief that one is deserving of punishment or is being punished (e.g. voices accusing one of sins or failures), nihilistic beliefs (delusions about the world ending or that one is going to be killed or is already dead), or bodily delusions (such as a belief that one is rotting away). Less often, depressed individuals may have delusions and hallucinations that are not related to depressive or destructive themes (e.g. belief that one's thoughts are being broadcast on the radio). Psychotic depression, even more than melancholic depressions, appear to be relatively stable over repeated episodes (Coryell et al., 1994; Sand and Harrow, 1994); that is, if a person has a psychotic depression their future episodes are also likely to show psychotic features.

(iv) **Postpartum Depression:** Many, perhaps most, women develop mild symptoms such as crying, insomnia, poor appetite, and mood variation in the period 3-7 days after giving birth. It is called "baby blues". These experiences are considered normal responses to the profound shifts in hormones. However, when a major depressive episode develops in the few weeks after delivery, it may be identified as major depression with postpartum onset. Generally speaking, the symptoms of postpartum depression are not different from symptoms of major depressives episode. Some studies have indicated that, if anything, postpartum depressions are generally milder than non-postpartum depressions (Whiffen and Gotlib, 1993). O'Hara and colleagues (1990) did not find any higher rates of postpartum depression than among demographically similar non-child bearing women. Moreover, several studies have indicated that postpartum status is probably not causally related to the depression. Instead, women who become depressed after childbirth are likely to have had previous emotional problems and vulnerabilities, with their depression likely the result of the stresses of having a child or marital difficulties (Gotlib, et al., 1991; O'Hara, et al., 1991). Women who do develop postpartum depression appear to be at increased risk for developing future depressive episodes, as indicated in a 41/2 year follow-up (Philipps and O'Hara, 1991).

Classification Used in Research

Some other classifications of depression used in research include:

(i) St. Louis Feigher Criteria: These criteria developed by Feigher et al., (1972) based on a distinction between 'primary' and 'secondary' depression as the central theme. This distinction is drawn on the basis of nature, history and antecedents of the disorder in a patient. When depression occurs in a patient with history of any other pre-existing psychiatric illness, it is termed as 'secondary' depression; while depression in the absence of such a history is 'primary'.

(ii) Catego: Catego is based on the 9th version of the present state examination (PSE) developed by Wing et al., (1974). Catego describes three classes of depression, namely,

(1) Class DT (or depressive psychosis),
(2) Class R (or retarded depression), and
(3) Class N (or neurotic depression).

It also describes four syndromes of depression, namely depressive delusions and hallucinations, simple depression, special symptoms of depression, and , other symptoms of depression.

(iii) Research Diagnostic Criteria (RDC): Developed by Spitzer, Endicott and Robins (1978), RDC lists the various diagnostic categories of depression under two broad headings namely major depressive disorder and minor depressive disorder, on the basis of severity of symptomatology. Although the major depressive disorder has about 12 sub-types, they are not mutually exclusive. The minor depressive disorder has two sub-types.

The RDC follows endogenous-reactive, psychotic-neurotic distinction in the classification of depression. It is a precursor to the DSM-III, DSM-III-R and DSM-IV systems, and the resemblance is obvious. It has been extensively used in research in the past.

(iv) Winokur's Familial System: Winokur (1979) has classified unipolar primary depression into the following categories:

(1) Familial Pure Depressive Disease (FPDD), where there is a family history of depression.
(2) Depressive Spectrum Disease, where there is a family history of alcoholism or sociopath but no family history of depression.
(3) Sporadic Depressive Disease, where there is no history of depression, alcoholism or sociopath.

Diagnosis of Depression

The first diagnostic distinction to be made is the difference between unipolar depression and bipolar disorder. Unipolar depression includes only depressive conditions occurring in the absence of current or past mania or hypomania. Mania and Hypomania (mild mania) are episodes of abnormal elevations of activity level, self-esteem, mood and other features that are in many ways the opposite of depression. Individuals who have cycles of both depression and mania/hypomania are considered to have bipolar affective disorder, which is a chronic problem of recurrent symptoms, often marked only by extreme mood swings but even by psychotic experiences including delusions and hallucinations. Even though their depressions may be indistinguishable from those of people who have only the severe unipolar form of the disorder, individual with bipolar disorder are considered to have an etiologically different disorder with a different course, and require different types of treatment. Hence, it is very important to evaluate meticulously not only the current symptoms but also the past history of mood disorders, keeping in mind that research has found that about 10.0% or more of initially depressed people go on to develop bipolar episodes (Coryell et al., 1995).

Bipolar I disorder includes a history of episodes of depression and mania while depression with history of hypomania is called Bipolar II disorder. Bipolar II is relatively more difficult to detect if the hypersomnia is more subtle or brief. An additional diagnostic problem is that sometimes there is no history of previous mania or hypermania but the person is nonetheless suffering from bipolar disorder. It has been demonstrated in longitudinal research that approximately 15.0% of individuals initially diagnosed with "unipolar" depression eventually 'switch' to bipolar disorder with the eventual display of manic/hypomanic episodes. The study of Akishal et al., 1995; and Coryell et al., 1995 also indicated that about 4.0% depressive patients converted to Bipolar I disorder overtime, and 8.6% converted to Bipolar II disorder.

Major Depressive Disorder

Box 1.1 displays the diagnostic criteria for major depressive disorder, according to DSMIV, and Box 1.3 (3.1) displays the very similar criteria in the International Classification of Diseases and related health problems (10th ed.) (ICD-10; World

Health Organization, 1993). For the diagnosis of major depressive disorder the individual must experience the symptoms for all or most of the time for at least two weeks. Also, in order to be diagnosed, the episode must be clinically significant in terms of causing distress or impaired functioning in the person's typical social or occupational roles.

Dysthymic Disorder

Box 1.2 displays the diagnostic criteria for Dysthymic Disorder, according to DSMIV, and Box 1.3 (3.2) also displays the very similar criteria in the International Classification of Diseases and related health problems (10th ed.) (ICD-10; World Health Organization, 1993). Dysthymic disorder would be diagnosed if symptoms persisted for at least two years (although there might be brief periods of normal mood lasting not more than 2 months). Additionally, in order to be diagnosed, dysthymic disorder must be seen to cause significant distress or disruption in the person's significant areas of functioning.

Diagnosis of Depression in Children and Adolescents

There are three key issues about the diagnosis of depression in youngsters. One is that the same criteria used for adults can be applied and that the essential features of the depressive syndrome are as recognizable in children as in adults (Carlson and Cantwell, 1980; Mitchell et al., 1988). Second, because children's externalizing or disruptive behaviours tend to attract more attention or are more readily expressed, compared to internal, subjective suffering, depression is sometimes overlooked. It may not be recognized, or it might not be assessed. Childhood depression has a high level of co-existing disorders, especially involving conduct problems and other disruptive behaviours; such patterns give rise to the erroneous belief that depression is 'masked.' Third, there are a few features of the syndrome of depression, such as irritable mood, that are more likely to be typical of children than of adults, leading to age-specific modifications of the diagnostic criteria. Major depression, therefore, would be diagnosed with adult

Box 1.1: Criteria for Major Depressive Disorder

A. Five (or more) of the following symptoms have to be present during the same 2-week period and represent a change from previous functioning; at least one of the symptoms is either (1) depressed mood or (2) loss of interest or pleasure.

1. Depressed mood for most of the day, nearly every day, as indicated by either subjective report (e.g., feels sad or empty) or observation made by others (e.g. appears tearful). In children and adolescents, can be irritable mood.
2. Markedly diminished interest or pleasure in all, or almost all, activities most of the day, nearly every day (as indicated by either subjective account or observation made by others).
3. Significant weight loss when not dieting or weight gain (e.g. a change of more than 5.0% of body weight in a month), or decrease or increase in appetite nearly every day. In children, consider failure to make expected weight gains.
4. Insomnia or hypersomnia nearly every day.
5. Psychomotor agitations or retardation nearly every day (observable by others, not merely subjective feeling of restlessness or being slowed down).
6. Fatigue or loss of energy nearly every day.
7. Feelings of worthlessness or excessive or inappropriate guilt (which may be delusional) nearly every day (not merely self-reproach or guilt about being sick).
8. Diminished ability to think or concentrate, or indecisiveness, nearly every day (either by subjective account or as observed by others).
9. Recurrent thoughts of death (not just fear of dying), recurrent suicidal ideation without a specific plan, or a suicide attempt or a specific plan for committing suicide.

B. The symptoms do not meet criteria for a Mixed Episode.

C. The symptoms are not due to the direct physiological effects of a substance (e.g. a drug of abuse, a medication) or a general medical condition (e.g. hypothyroidism).

D. The symptoms are not better accounted for by Bereavement, i.e., after the loss of a loved one, the symptoms persist for longer than 2 months or are characterized by marked functional impairment, morbid preoccupation with worthlessness, suicidal ideation, psychotic symptoms, or psychomotor retardation.

Box 1.2: Diagnostic Criteria for Dysthymic Disorder

A. Depressed mood for most of the day, for more days than not, as indicated either by subjective account or observation by others, for at least 2 years. In children and adolescents, mood can be irritable and duration must be at least 1 year.

B. Presence, while depressed, of two (or more) of the following:

(1) Poor appetite or overeating
(2) Insomnia or hypersomnia
(3) Low energy or fatigue
(4) Low self-esteem
(5) Poor concentration or difficulty making decision
(6) Feelings of hopelessness

C. During the 2-years period (1 year for children or adolescents) of the disturbance, the person has never been without the symptoms in Criteria A and B for more than 2 months at a time.

D. No Major Depressive Episode has occurred during the first 2 years of the disturbance (1 year for children and adolescents); i.e., the disturbance is not better accounted for by chronic Major Depressive Disorder, or Major Depressive Disorder, in Partial Remission.

E. There has never been a Manic Episode, a Mixed Episode, or a Hypomanic Episode, and criteria have never been met for Cyclothymic Disorder.

F. The disturbance does not occur exclusively during the course of a chronic Psychotic Disorder, such as Schizophrenia or Delusional Disorder.

G. The symptoms are not due to the direct physiological effect of a substance (e.g., drug of abuse, a medication) or a general medical condition (e.g. hypothyroidism).

H. The symptoms cause clinically significant distress or impairment in social, occupational, or other important areas of functioning.

Box 1.3: Diagnostic Criteria for Depressive Disorders (ICD-10, World Health Organization, 1993)

Note: General diagnostic criteria and clinical features are specified, but the following are the more precisely defined diagnostic criteria for research (for depressive episode and dysthymia)

3.1 Depressive Episode

A. Symptoms must be present for at least weeks; the person did not meet criteria for mania or hypomania at any time.

B. (a) Depressed mood most of the day and almost every day, uninfluenced by circumstances,
   (b) Loss of interest or pleasure in activities that are normally pleasurable,
   (c) Increased fatigability or decreased energy.

C. (a) Loss of confidence or self-esteem,
   (b) Unreasonable feelings of self-reproach or excessive and inappropriate guilt,
   (c) Recurrent thoughts of death or suicide, or any suicidal behaviour,
   (d) Complaints or evidence of diminished ability to think or concentrate, such as indecisiveness or vacillation,
   (e) Change in psychomotor activity, with agitation or retardation (either subjective or objective),
   (f) Sleep disturbance of any type,
   (g) Change in appetite (decrease or increase) with corresponding weight change).

Note: Depressive episodes may be diagnosed as:

- **Mild** (at least 2 from B plus at least 2 from C, for a total of at least 4);
- **Moderate** (at least 2 from B plus, 3 or 4 from C, for a total of at least 6);
- **Severe depressive episode** without psychotic features (all 3 from B plus, at least 4 from C, for a total of at least 9-no hallucinations, delusions or depressive stupor).

3.2 Dysthymia

A. There must be a period of at least 2 years of constant or constantly recurring depressed mood; intervening periods of normal mood rarely last for longer than a few weeks; and there are no episodes of hypomania.

B. None, or very few, individual episodes within the 2 years period are sufficiently severe or long lasting to meet criteria for recurrent mild depressive disorder.

C. During at least some of the periods of depression at least 3 of the following should be present:
   (a) Reduced energy or activity,
   (b) Insomnia,
   (c) Loss of self-confidence or feelings of inadequacy,
   (d) Difficulty in concentrating,
   (e) Frequent tearfulness,
   (f) Loss of interest in or enjoyment of sex and other pleasurable activities,
   (g) Feeling of hopelessness or despair,
   (h) A perceived inability to cope with the routine responsibilities of everyday life,
   (i) Pessimism about the future or brooding over the past,
   (j) Social withdrawal,
   (k) Reduced talkativeness.

criteria as in Box 1.1 and 1.3(3.1), but permitting irritability instead of depressed mood. Dysthymia in children must persist at least for one year (in adults duration is at least two years). According to a recent study of dysthymic disorder in children, it differs from major depression primarily in the emphasis on gloomy thoughts and other negative affect, with fewer symptoms such as loss of interest, social withdrawal, fatigue, and reduced sleep and poor appetite (Kovacs et al., 1994).

Developmental considerations should be taken into account when assessing for depression in children. For instance, irritability may be substituted for depressed mood because it is recognized both that irritability is a common expression of distress in depressed youngsters and that young depressed children may not express subjective negative affect. Goodyer and Cooper (1993) found that 80.0% of their sample of 11-16 year-old girls with major depressive episode reported irritability, while Ryan et al., (1987) observed irritability or anger in 83.0% of a child and adolescent clinic sample.

Young depressed children, especially preschoolers and preadolescents, are unlikely to report subjective dysphoria and hopelessness, but instead "look" depressed in facial expression and posture (Carlson and Kashani, 1988; Ryan et al., 1987). In adolescence, by contrast, depressed mood is commonly reported by more than 90.0% of those with major depression

(Mitchell et al., 1988; Ryan et al., 1987). Also, younger depressed children are more likely to have physically unjustified or exaggerated somatic complaints (Kashani and Carlson, 1987; Ryan et al., 1987). In a community sample, depressive symptoms were more associated with physical complaints among 12-year-olds than they were for 17-year-olds (Kashani et al., 1989), Younger Children also show more irritability, uncooperativeness, apathy, and lack of interest (Kashani et al., 1986),

Two studies compared the symptoms of depressed youngsters and adults. Overall, several symptoms increase with age: loss of pleasure, psychomotor retardation, and diurnal variation, while several decrease with age: depressed appearance, physical complaints, and poor self-esteem (Carlosn and Kashani, 1988). Comparing combined child-adolescent groups with a sample of adults, Mitchell et al., (1988) found similar differences for self-esteem, somatic complaints, diurnal variation, and also found that adult depressed patients reported less guilt and more early morning awakening and weight loss than the depressed youngsters.

In addition to presentation of depressive symptoms, patterns of comorbid disorders are also likely to be somewhat different at different ages. For instance, depressed children and young adolescents are more likely than depressed older adolescents to display separation anxiety disorders (Fleming and Offord, 1990). Other kinds of anxiety disorders and disruptive behavioural disorders appear to co-exist with depression for both children and adolescents.

There are several other symptoms frequently seen in children and adolescents. Social withdrawal is common in both the groups. Excessive worrying and other anxiety symptoms are common, as are oppositional and conduct problems (Goodyer and Cooper, 1993; Mitchell et al., 1988) Indeed, the likelihood of comorbid anxiety and disruptive behaviour disorder diagnoses is very high i.e., 60.0-70.0%. Somatic symptoms and bodily complaints are also frequently associated with depression, as noted earlier, and problems with self-esteem—and in adolescent girls, distress over negative body image—are also common associated symptoms of depression (Allgood-Merten Lewinsohn, and Hops, 1990; Petersen, Sarigiani, and Kennedy, 1991).

Suicidal thoughts and attempts are among the diagnostic criteria for major depression. Suicidal ideation is quite common in depressed youngsters, occurring in about two-thirds of preschoolers, preadolescents, and adolescents (Kashani and Carlson, 1987; Mitchell et al., 1988; Ryan et al., 1987). Actual suicidal attempts occurred in 39.0% of the preadolescent and adolescent samples of Mitchell et al., (1988), with 6.0-12.0% of the Ryan et al., (1987) child and adolescent samples making moderate or severe attempts. These rates appear to be higher among depressed youngsters than among depressed adults.

Causal Factors of Depression

A specific causal factor of depression has not been found. However. the causative factors can artificially be divided into genetic factors, biochemical factors and psycho-social factors. The division is artificial because of the likelihood that the three realms interact among themselves. These etiological factors of depression are given below:

Genetic Factors

The genetic data strongly indicate that a significant factor in the development of depression is genetics. The methods of genetic research include family studies, adoption studies and twin studies.

(A) Family Studies: A number of studies of adult depressed probands have been conducted. Gershon (1990) reviewed ten such studies of unipolar depressed patients, and found that the rates of depression in first-degree relatives ranged between 7.0% and 30.0%—considerably higher than in the general population. In the Collaborative Depression Study of nearly 900 patients and controls, the rate of severe major depression involving hospitalization, incapacitation, or psychosis was 10.4% in first-degree relatives of unipolar probands, compared with 4.9% of controls' relatives (Winokur et al., 1995).

Klein et al., (1995) found that dysthymia was significantly more common in the relatives of dysthymic patients than in either major depressed or normal comparisons, but that these families also displayed elevated rates of major depression. Both dysthymia and major depression in patients were also associated with elevated rates of personality disorders in relatives, although the association was especially strong for dysthymic patients.

(B) Adoption Studies: Adoption studies have also produced data that support the genetic basis for the inheritance of depression. According to adoption studies children of depressed parents appear to be at increased risk for developing depression as well as other disorders. Many studies found that about 50.0% to 80.0% of children of depressed parents display a diagnosable disorder during childhood or adolescence, about 50.0% of the offspring display depressive disorders but the full array of conduct, anxiety, and substance abuse disorders may also be present. (Weissman et al., 1987; Gotlib and Lee, 1990; Klein et al., 1988). While early onset of disorder may be an indicator of genetically transmitted dysfunction, most of the offspring studies also indicate that the children in such families not only inherit whatever biological factors may contribute to psychiatric disorders, but they also "inherit" a variety of psychosocial disturbances such as dysfunctional child rearing and highly stressful family environments (Hammen, 1991a).

(C) Twin Studies: In view of the difficulty in drawing conclusions about specifically genetic transmission from family patterns of disorder, many investigators have turned to twin study methods. Since identical (monozygotic) twins share 100% of their genes, they should be more similar to each other in the expression of a disorder (concordance) than would twins who are not identical (dizygotic) and who share an average of 50.0% of their genes. Indeed, earlier twin studies have generally indicated approximately 4 times higher concordance rates in monozygotic than dizygotic twins (65.0% to 14.0%) according to a review by Nurnberger and Gershon (1984).

McGuffin et al., (1996) conducted a study on 214 twin pairs through probands and revealed that concordance for lifetime major depression was 46.0% for monozygotic twins, compared with 20.0% for dizygotic twins, and both rates were substantially higher than lifetime depression in the general population. McGuffin et al., (1996) concluded that genetic factors play a moderate role in family patterns of depression, and also suggested that genetics may be particularly important in recurrent depression with endogenous (melancholic) features.

Kendler et al., (1992) also tested the genetic versus shared environment hypothesis in their study of 1033 female twin pairs from the community-based Virginia Twin Registry. Using various diagnostic criteria to define depression, concordance between monozygotic (MZ) twins was higher than for dizygotic (DZ) twins and both groups had higher rates of depression than did the general population. Kendler et al., (1993) also found 27.0% concordance for MZ twins and 17.6% concordance for DZ twins. Plomin et al., (1997) also reviewed evidence from five studies showing that monozygotic co-twins of a twin with unipolar major depression are about two to four times as likely to develop major depression as are dizygotic co-twins of a depressed twin.

Biochemical Factors

Every human being has a unique biochemical makeup. Whether or not a person will experience depression (or other neurological disorders) depends largely on the amount of certain brain chemicals and how they interact in the central nervous system (CNS). The different biochemical factors of depression are:

(A) Neurotransmitters

Starting in the 1960s, the view that depression may arise from disruptions in the delicate balance of neurotransmitter substances that regulate and mediate the activity of the brain's nerve cells, or neurons, has received a great deal of attention. Neurotransmitters are, of course, the "chemical messengers" by which neurons communicate and link the regions and functions of various parts of the brain.

Historically, there has been considerable interest in the potential role of monoamine neurotransmitters (especially sertonin, norepinephrine (noradrenaline), and dopamine) in mood disorders. The monomine neurotransmitters were known to be especially important in the functioning of the limbic system of the brain (amygdala, hippocampus, hypothalamus, and related structures of the "old brain"), areas that play a major role in the regulation of drives (e.g. appetite) and emotion. Limbic system neurotransmitter pathways link this region with other parts of the brain, and also, through the hypothalamus, exert control over the endocrine and autonomic nervous systems (Shelton et al., 1991).

In the 1950s, several medications were observed either to cause or decrease depression, and it became known that they had their effects on the central monoamine neurotransmitters. For example, tricyclic antidepressants such as imipramine were found to block the synaptic reuptake of amines into the presynapatic neurons, thus increasing their availability (Mc Neal and Cimbolic, 1986). Based on the apparent monoaminergic effects of drugs,

Schildkraut (1965) articulated a catecholamine model of affective disorders that claimed depression results from insufficiencies of the monoamine neurotransmitters. Siever and Davis (1985) proposed a dysregulation model of neurotransmitters in depression, hypothesising that instability, desynchronisation, and abnormal reactivity in the monoamine neurotransimitter system causes depression.

(B) Neuroendocrine Functioning

The monoaminergic neurotransmitters play a crucial role in the various brain functions, including the limbic system. The hypothalamus exerts control over the endocrine and autonomic nervous systems. There has been considerable interest in the role of such processes in depression. For instance, in the search for differences between depressed and non-depressed persons, one of the most consistent findings concerns cortisol and related functioning of the hypothalamic-pituitary-adrenal (HPA) axis. The HPA axis is a neuroendocrine system involving complex interconnections between the brain, certain hormones, and various organs. It is centrally involved in the body's normal reactions to stress. When the person perceives stress, under the control of various neurotransmitters such as norepinephrine, serotonin, gamma-aminobutyric acid (GABA), and acetylcholine, the hypothalamus in the brain synthesizes the hormone CRF (Corticoticotropin-Releasing Factor), which then stimulates the anterior pituitary gland resulting in the synthesis and release of an adrenocorticotropic hormone (ACTH). ACTH then circulates to the adrenal glands, located on the kidneys, which produce cortisol. Cortisol is a key hormone in the sympathetic nervous system, resulting in a variety of forms of physical arousal and activation. The presence of cortisol in the blood then inhibits further production of ACTH and corticotropin-releasing hormone (CRH). In normal people, therefore, this homeostatic mechanism prevents excessive or prolonged physiological arousal. Numerous studies have found elevated levels of cortisol in acutely depressed people compared to nondepressed (as well as increased levels of CRF). When the person is no longer depressed, cortisol levels return to normal.

(C) Sleep and Other Biological Rhythms

(i) Sleep Disturbance Pattern: Sleep is characterized by five stages that occur in a relatively invariant sequence throughout the night (stages 1 to 4 of non-REM sleep and REM sleep). REM (Rapid Eye Movement) sleep is characterized by rapid eye movements and dreaming, as well as other bodily changes.

A number of studies have found disruption in sleep patterns, both behavioural and as measured by electroencephalogram (EEG) recordings. For example, over the past 25 years, three sleep pattern abnormalities have been well documented in depressed patients. One is a sleep continuity problem, including difficulty falling asleep or staying asleep, and waking up early. These abnormalities are present in about 80.0% of people in a major depression, although they are not limited to depressive conditions (Ford and Kamerow, 1989, Kupfer and Thase, 1983). A Second abnormality is decreased slow-wave (delta) sleep, as recorded by brain-wave activity during sleep (Reynolds and Kupfer, 1987). This pattern is most apparent in depressives with so-called endogenous (melancholic) features. The third abnormality is alterations in the nature and timing of Rapid Eye Movement (REM) sleep. Thase et al., (1995) noted that normal people experience the onset of the first REM period about 1 to 2 hours after falling asleep, with subsequent REM periods increasing in length and intensity occurring at about 90-minute intervals. About 50.0% of depressed patients, by contrast, have shortened REM latencies—that is, they begin REM sleep in less than 60 minutes, and increased REM activity with a shift of REM activity into the first few hours of sleep (REM density). Disturbed REM sleep may be a marker of a particularly pernicious form of depression, with an increased risk of relapse (Reynolds and Kupfer, 1987).

Several studies have suggested that sleep abnormalities are relatively stable, and remain unchanged when the depression remits (Giles et al., 1993). Thase et al., (1994) examined the sleep patterns of unmedicated male patients undergoing psychotherapy. They found that with clinical improvement, the sleep profiles showed a significant reduction in REM sleep density. However, there were no changes in reduced REM latency or slow-wave sleep. These results suggest either that the latter are stable traits—possibly serving as markers for future risk of relapse or possibly they do return to normal levels with the passage of time.

It is of interest to note that abnormal sleep patterns may be familial, perhaps indicating a genetically transmitted marker or process of vulnerability. Giles, et al., (1992) found correlated patterns of sleep abnormalities in youngsters and their parents in families with depression. Lauer et al., (1995) studied sleep patterns of 54 healthy adults who were considered at risk for mood disorders because a close relative had displayed reduced slow-wave sleep and increased REM densities, the authors suggest that such patterns may mark a vulnerability for future depression.

(ii) **Circadian Rhythms:** The abnormal patterns of circadian rhythm functions such as cortisol secretion and sleep disturbances have suggested a dysfunction of some type. One hypothesis is that there is a disorganization or desynchronisation of different cycles in relation to each other. Normally, REM patterns and cortisol fluctuate in synchrony with the sleep—wake cycle. Early morning awakening, diurnal variation, and the abnormalities noted have suggested a "phase advance" of the REM and cortisol secretion circadian rhythms in relation to the sleep—wake cycle. The desynchrony results in biological disturbances causing the symptoms of depression. Interestingly, sleep deprivation has been shown to reduce depression, at least temporarily, possibly by bringing the circadian rhythms back into alignment with each other (Wu and Bunney, 1990).

(iii) **Sunlight and Seasons:** Another kind of rhythm abnormality or disturbance may be seen in sub-type of unipolar depression known as *seasonal affective disorder*. This type of patients seem to be responsive to the total quantity of available light in the environment (Oren and Rosenthal, 1992) becoming depressed in the fall and winter and normalizing in spring and winter.

(D) Brain Structure and Functioning

Individuals who sustain injuries or strokes in the frontal part of the brain have often been observed to display depression. One condition, post *stroke depression,* has been estimated to affect 30.0% to 50.0% of individuals after acute stroke.

Examination of the association between stroke location and presence of depression has suggested that the frontal regions and left side of the brain are especially critical, particularly the left frontal region, but the right posterior region of the frontal lobes may also be important in post stroke depression (Starkstein and Robinson, 1991). The frontal lobes control not only the higher intellectual functions such as planning and judgment, but are also a major regulatory component of the limbic system. Starkstein and Robinson (1991) speculate that stroke induced damage to the biogenic amine pathways that connect the frontal regions to the limbic system may account for the symptomatology of depression.

Building on such observations and hypotheses, investigators have looked at the possibility of brain abnormalities in depressed patients. Neuroimaging studies, for example, have provided some evidence of structural abnormalities in the frontal regions of unipolar patients, particularly severely depressed patients (Powell and Miklowitz, 1994). Coffey et al., (1993) used magnetic resonance imaging (MRI) analysis to demostrate that depressed patients had lower frontal lobe volume than did controls, although there were no temporal lobe volume than did controls, although there were no temporal lobe volume differences.

Another method for assessing frontal lobe functioning is electrophysiological (EEG) recording. Davidson and his colleague (Henriques and Davidson, 1990) reviewed evidence from various sources, concluding that depression is associated with a decrease in either left frontal or right posterior activation. They demonstrated left frontal hypoactivation in a sample of

15 unipolar depressed patients compared with normal controls (Henriques and Davidson, 1991)

Henriques and Davidson (1990) evaluated individuals who previously had experienced a major depressive episode but who were now non-depressed, and compared them with never-depressed individuals. The former depressives were found to have the predicted reduced activation in the left frontal and right posterior cortical regions. Devidson speculates that deficits in left anterior activation reflect deficits in an "approach" system, and that individuals who display this type of frontal EEG asymmetry are more vulnerable to negative affective states including depression given sufficient environmental stress.

(E) Fluctuating Hormone Levels

In women, fluctuating hormone levels can contribute to depression. Conditions linked to hormones in women are:

- **Premenstrual Syndrome:** Approximately 3.0%-8.0% of women in their reproductive years are affected with premenstrual syndrome (PMS) during the week or so before their menstrual period. PMS is characterized by depressed mood, mood swings, irritability, and tension or anxiety. It lessens with the onset of the menstrual period each month.
- **Postpartum Depression:** Postpartum depression actually refers to three distinct phenomena *postpartum blues* occur in a substantial percentage of women in the first few days after birth. Symptoms of crying, sadness, and upset are short-lived and rarely treated. They are thought to be consequences of the dramatic drops in estrogen and progesterone levels that occur at birth. Thus, this reaction is normal, and does not resemble the clinical condition of depression. *Postpartum major depression*, on the other hand, meets criteria for major depression and may occur in 10.0-15.0% of women after birth. Since only a minority of women experiences such depression, they are clearly not an inevitable response

to hormonal changes. In general, women who do experience such depression display psychosocial difficulties and prior histories of depression (Gotlib et al., 1991, O' Hara et al., 1991). The depression may also be related to large changes in hormones and cortisol (Weissman and Olfson, 1995). Women who develop postpartum depression are at increased risk for developing depressive episodes in future.

- **Depression in Menopause:** Menopausal depression was once attributed to middle-aged women feeling sad over the loss of their childbearing capabilities (the loss of their "youth" or "femininity"), and the loss of their grown children (the "empty nest"). There is no evidence that this is true. In fact, evidence suggests that for some women, menopause and the "empty nest" may signify a new freedom in their lives to pursue long-delayed interests and devote more time to their own needs.

However, hormonal fluctuations in menopause are real, and some women suffer from mood swings, fatigue, and depression. Hormone replacement therapy (HRT) can lift mood and fatigue among women who are medically able and who choose to take HRT.

Psychosocial Factors

Most forms of psychological disorder affect individual's interpersonal lives, impairing their social functioning by altering interpersonal behaviours and the quality of relating to others. Depression is no exception because the symptoms of depression interfere with normal relationships. But even more importantly, several perspectives about the causes of depression emphasize the role of relatedness to others as a fundamental contributing factor. There is no single interpersonal perspective on depression; instead there are diverse topics of study, such as premorbid personality factor, family functioning, attachment, marital adjustment, loss and bereavement, and the effects of stressful interpersonal events, and social skills. Difficulties in social relatedness have been variously viewed as concomitants of being in a depressed state, consequences of depression that have negative "side effects", and as fundamental causal factors in depression.

(A) Premorbid Personality Factor

No single personality trait or type uniquely predisposes one to depression. All humans, of whatever personality pattern, can and do become depressed under appropriate circumstances, however certain personality types such as oral—dependent, obsessive-compulsive, hysterical—may be at greater risk for depression than are antisocial, paranoid, and other personality types who use projection and other externalizing defense mechanism.

(B) Early Childhood Experiences

Many researches indicate that the quality of early life experiences in the family may contribute to depression. The quality of the attachment bond, the experience of critical, rejecting, or over controlling parenting and disrupted family life appear to set the stage for depression. Children exposed to such experiences may become depressed, while adults who experience such events in childhood may be vulnerable to depressive reactions when faced with triggering experiences.

(i) Attachment and Depression: Both *psychodynamic and social learning* theory models of human development emphasize the importance of experiences in early childhood in the family environment. When those experiences are dysfunctional or when the child lacks critical experiences such as a close bond with a stable caretaker, he or she may develop in maladaptive ways. Both of these models hypothesize that depression might be a form of psychopathology resulting from certain unique family experiences.

John Bowlby (1978; 1981) has articulated a model of the importance of early attachment bonds between the infant and the caretaker, which has implications not only for depression, but also for key elements of individual personality and adaptive functioning.

Kobak et al., (1991) and Hammen et al., (1995) also showed that adolescents were more likely to become depressed following stressful life events if they had more insecure attachment representations of their parents. A study of clinically depressed women patients found that they reported significantly less attachment to their mothers than did non-psychiatric controls (Rosenfarb et al., 1994).

Taken together, the few attachment studies support a link between quality of early childhood attachment and vulnerability to depressive reactions. In general, the retrospective studies are fairly consistent: depressed adults report more adverse relationship with their parents during childhood. Andrews and Brown (1988) found that women who became clinically depressed following occurrence of major life events were more likely to report lack of adequate parental care or hostility from their mothers, compared to those who did not become depressed (Brown and Harris, 1993). In reviewing the extensive literature on depressed individuals' recollections of parents, Gerlsma et al., (1990) concluded that parental childrearing styles that included low affection and more control (overprotection) were especially consistently related to depression.

Recently, Research shows that such parental styles were not only associated with the occurrence of depression, but also with its course features. For instance, Lizardi et al., (1995) examined the childhood experiences of patients who had diagnoses of early onset dysthymic disorder, and found that they were significantly more likely to have experienced negative relations with their parents than were comparison groups of normal controls or those with major depressive episodes. In another study, severity of symptoms, as well as highly negative cognitions, were particularly associated with adverse family experience including harsh, rigid control, overprotection, or sexual assault (Rose et al., 1994). Gotlib et al., (1988) examined the reports of women with or without postpartum depression concerning their own parents' childrearing styles. They found that the depressed women reported less maternal and paternal care and more maternal overprotection. Also, a further study of postpartum depressed women found that negative perceptions of parents predicted the onset of depression during the postpartum period, and more negative perceptions predicted slower recovery (Gotlib et al., 1991).

Although the research links depression with somewhat general parental styles reflection negativity (criticism, low affection or care, over controlling), some investigators suggest that different types of depression might be associated with more specific patterns. Blatt and Homann (1992), adopting a psychodynamic object-relations model of depression, argued that insecure attachment characterized by anxiety and neediness would lead to a depression focused on dependency and concerns about abandonment ('anaclitic' depression characterized by helplessness and weakness). Insecure attachment characterized by an avoidant or dismissive reaction toward others, on the other hand, would lead to a depression focused on issues of self-worth, self-criticism, and achievement (an 'introjective' depression, characterized by feelings of inferiority, failure, and guilt. According to Blatt and Homann (1992), introjectively depressed persons are likely to have had parents who set high standards, and are harshly critical, intrusive, and controlling in and attempt to get their children to meet their high expectations. As a result, the child constantly berates herself or himself, and attacks the self as worthless.

(ii) **Early Loss and Depression:** Numerous studies have tested the theory that depression is often caused by loss of a parent in early childhood, presumably creating a vulnerability to become depressed later in life if a real or threatened loss of a loved one reactivates the despair of the early loss. Some researchers have viewed that not only early parental loss but lack of quality and inconsistent care for the child also leads to depression (Bifulco, et al., 1987; Harris, et al., 1986). Harris and colleagues hypothesize that the adult women in their studies who lost a parent in childhood and were then subjected to poor care were likely to experience lowered self-esteem. Later on, exposure to highly stressful life events, therefore, might cause a generalized sense of hopelessness, hence depression, in those with low self-esteem.

(iii) **Specific Childhood Stressors and Vulnerability to Depression:** In addition to loss and inadequate parenting, several studies point to the impact of particular childhood stressors. A large-scale epidemiological study of community residents who met criteria for major depression found that several childhood adversities (parental drinking, parental mental illness, family violence, parental marital problems, deaths of mother or father, and lack of a close relationship with an adult) were predictive of onset of depression. Three early adversities, parental mental illness, violence, and parental divorce, were significantly predictive of recurrence of depression (Kessler and Magee, 1993).

Several Studies have indicated that the experience of childhood physical and sexual abuse may be associated with later depression (and other disorders) (Andrews et al., 1990; Brown and Andeson, 1991; Brown and Harris, 1993). Abuse was especially associated with recurrent depression. Similar findings were reported for those with early onset of dysthymia, which by definition is a chronic disorder for with men and women, childhood sexual assault, was particularly related to likelihood of adult disorders including depression (Burnam et al., 1988).

(C) Marital Problem

There is a large body of research showing an association between marital status or quality and depression. Studies of marital couples are one, which in clinically depressed have shown relationally negative interaction patterns marked by hostility, tension, difficulty resolving conflict, and reports of marital difficulties associated with depression (Fadden et at., 1987). Gotlib and Hammen (1992) suggest that intimate/happy marital relationship with the spouse is protection against depression, even in the face of major stressors. On the other hand, marital distress can lead to depressive episode or marital conflict and criticism can prolong depression or precipitate relapses.

(D) Cognitive Model of Depression

According to Beck's cognitive theory of depression (Beck, 1967) there are certain depressogenic schemas or dysfunctional beliefs, which are developed during childhood and adolescence as a function of one's experiences with parents or with significant others (teachers, peers etc.). Children who lose parent or who have poor parenting are prone to develop depressogenic schemas. The dysfunctional schemas or beliefs make a person vulnerable to depression if he/she encounters certain significant stressors. Once activated the dysfunctional beliefs trigger automatic thoughts that in turn produce depressive symptoms, which further fuel the depressive automatic thoughts.

Other Factors

Other factors that can lead to depression include:

- Alcohol or drug abuse.

- Use of certain medications, such as steroids and some blood pressure medications.
- Underlying general medical conditions that can cause depressive symptoms, such as hypothyroidism (underactive thyroid gland), chronic fatigue syndrome, and others.
- "Burnout," a depletion of mental and physical energy usually stemming from prolonged overwork and/or an overload of demands and obligations placed upon an individual.

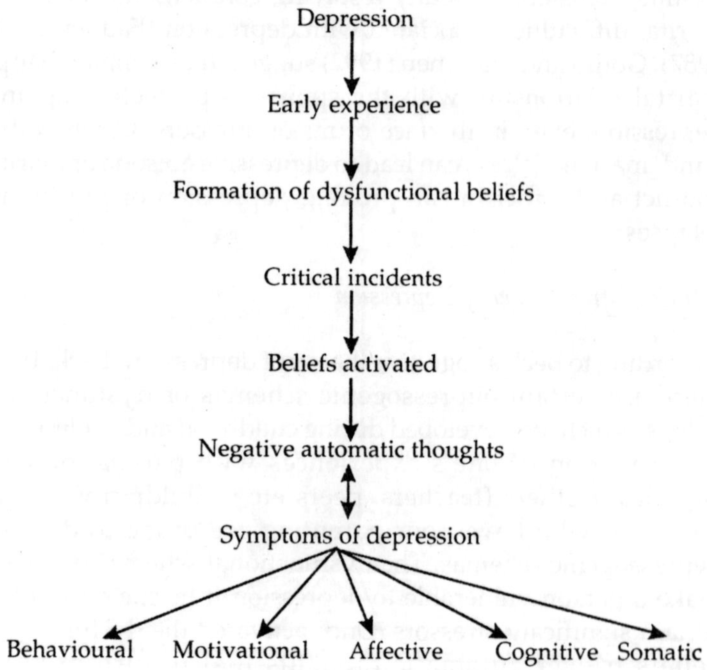

Model 1.1: Beck's Cognitive Model of Depression

Consequences of Depression

Depression can be devastating to family relationships, friendships, and the ability to work or to go to school. It affects the quality of life, productiveness of an individual. The depressed person faces problem to cope everywhere—at home, at school, in friend circle, in social occasions or even at road. At depression's worst, the afflicted person may spend endless hours in bed; often find it difficult to perform even minimal tasks such as bathing or getting dressed.

Depression cause pain and suffering not only to those who are the victims of this deadly disease, but also to those who care about them. Their persistent depressed mood, irritation, agitation, constant lethargy, not caring to others, lack of sense of responsibility, pessimistic thoughts and suicidal ideation make others also irritated and sad. Family members do not get any means to make the suffered person's mind happy, to bring him/her into the normal stream of life. Such mental condition of their nearest and dearest one makes them also unhappy, helpless, hopeless and anxious. Initially the family members respond to the depressed person with concern and compassion, but their reaction eventually turn to dejection and hostility because of the aversiveness of the disease.

Impaired Interpersonal Relationship

Depressed people not only have interpersonal problems, but their own behaviour also seems to make these problems worse. A depressed person may induce depressed feeling and negative affect in others (Howes et al., 1985; Joiner et al., 1995) and may make a non-depressed person less willing to interact again with the depressed person.

Depression negatively affects marital relationships. Sometimes poor marriages cause depression but often it is depression that causes marital problems. Depressed people and their spouses tend to perceive their interactions as marked by tension and hostility, which often persist even after the depressed spouse recovers. The effects of depression are diverse, probably including irritability, withdrawal, dependency, and other symptoms. Also, of course, depressed spouses are often viewed as a great burden, causing worry, reducing the sharing of pleasurable activities, failing to respond to encouragement and support.

Depression causes significant impairment in parent-child relationship. The effect of depression in one family extend to infants, children and adolescent, as well. Parental depression puts children at high risk for many problems, but especially for depression (Murray et al., 1996). For adolescent girls, it also increases risk of conduct problems (Davies and Windle, 1997). Depressed mother often wish to be good parents, and are troubled by their difficulties. Nonetheless depression takes an enormous tool on their energy, interest, patience, and mood—all of which doubtless impair their abilities to sustain positive, supportive, and attentive relationships with their children. Not only this depressed youngsters also have negative interactions with their parents.

Mortality due to Depression

Depression is one of the few psychological disorders that can be said to be fatal. Suicide now ranks among the ten leading causes of death in most Western countries. In the United States it is the eighth or ninth leading cause of death, with current estimates of more than 30,000 suicides each year (Silverman, 1997).

The risk of suicide—taking one's own life—is a significant factor in all depressive states. Of all the consequences, suicide is, of course, the starkest consequences of the individual's feeling of hopelessness and debility. Although it is obvious that people also commit suicide for reasons other than depression, depressed people are 20 times more likely to commit suicide than non-depressed people (Clark, 1995). About 10.0-15.0% of individuals with a diagnosis of major depressive disorder eventually kill themselves (Maris et al., 1992). Depression is also associated with increased mortality due to accidents and medical problems.

Treatment of Depression

Depression is a serious, potentially life threatening medical illness, and both the patients and their families deserve much support. Most clinicians and researchers believe that combined psychotherapy and pharmacotherapy is the most effective treatment for depressive disorder. Combined therapy helps a patient to develop more stable, long-range adjustment.

Considerable evidence also suggests that certain forms of psychotherapy for depression, alone or in combination of pharmacotherapy, significantly decrease the likelihood of relapse within a two-year follow up period (Hollon et al., 1996).

Pharmacotherapy

Anti-depressant medications are widely used and effective treatment for depression. Existing anti-depressants influence the functioning of certain chemicals in the brain called neurotransmitters. The newer medications, such as the selective serotonin reuptake inhibitors (SSRIs), tend to have fewer side effects than the older drugs, which include tricyclic anti-depressants (TCAs) and monoamine oxidase inhibitors (MAOIs).

Electroconvulsive Therapy (ECT)

ECT is often used in case of severely depressed patients as anti-depressants often take three to four weeks to produce significant improvement. ECT is currently administered under medically safe conditions, in which patients are first given sedatives, muscle relaxants or other agents to control potentially damaging physical side effects. The person receiving ECT does not consciously experience the electrical stimulus.

ECT is useful, particularly for individual whose depression is severe or life threatening or who don't respond to other pharmacological treatment (Weiner and Coffey, 1988). ECT is considered as the treatment of choice for the elderly who often either cannot take anti-depressant medications or who don't respond well to them (Niederehe and Schneider, 1998). When selection criteria of this form of treatment are carefully observed, a complete remission of symptoms occurs after 6 to 12 treatments (with two or three per week being typical), meaning that a majority of severely depressed patients can be vastly better in two to four weeks (Gitlin, 1996).

Psychotherapy

Although psychoanalytic approaches were the predominant mode of treatment for depression in the early to middle part of this century, now many types of psychotherapy based on a variety of concepts are in use.. Psychotherapeutic approaches have been developed specifically for depression that aim to correct specific manifestations, including cognition, behaviour and affect.

(A) Cognitive Behaviour Therapy (CBT)

CBT stems from four major theories: Psychoanalytic theory, phenomenological philosophy, cognitive psychology and behavioural psychology. Aaron Beck, the originator of Cognitive Behavioural Therapy (CBT), developed a comprehensive, structured theory of depression. According to this theory depression is associated with negative thought patterns, specific distorted schemas and cognitive errors or faulty information processing. Such cognitive dysfunctions form the core of depression while affective and physical changes and other associated features of depression are in consequences.

CBT focuses on the cognitive distortions postulated to be present in major depressive disorder. Such distortions include selective attention to the negative aspects of circumstances and unrealistically morbid inferences about consequences.

The goal of CBT is to change the way a person thinks and subsequently, to alleviate the depressive syndrome and prevent its reoccurrence. This is accomplished by helping the patient (a) identify and test negative cognitions, (b) develop alternative more flexible schemas, and (c) rehearse both new cognitive and new behavioural responses.

CBT is a short-term, structured therapy that involves active collaboration between the patient and the therapist toward achieving set goals. It is oriented toward current problems and their resolution. It is an effective treatment for many out patients with major depressive disorder. This therapy is particularly effective among mild to moderately depressed patients and may be less effective than pharmacotherapy among more severely depressed patients.

(B) Interpersonal Therapy (IPT)

Interpersonal therapy, developed by Gerald Klerman, focuses on one or two of the patient's current interpersonal problems, using two assumptions: first current interpersonal problems are likely to have their roots in early dysfunctional relationships. Second, current interpersonal problems are likely to involved in precipitating or perpetuating the current depressive symptoms. The interpersonal therapy approach to depression involves three interacting components: Symptom formation, social and interpersonal experiences, and enduring personality patterns.

The goal of interpersonal therapy is to (i) reduce the patient's depressive symptoms and improve self-esteem, and (ii) help the patient to develop more effective strategies for dealing with current social and interpersonal relations.

The interpersonal therapy programme usually consists of 12 to 16 weekly sessions. The therapy is characterized by an active approach on the part of the therapist and by an emphasis on current issues and social functioning in the life of the patients. Intra-psychic phenomenon such as, defense mechanisms, or internal conflicts are not addressed. Discrete behaviours such as lack of assertiveness, social skills or distorted thinking may be addressed, but only in the context of their meaning or effect on interpersonal relationships.

(C) Behaviour Therapy

Behaviour therapy is an effective treatment modality for major depressive disorder. This therapy is based on the hypothesis that maladaptive behavioural patterns result in a person's receiving little positive feedback from society and perhaps outright rejection. By addressing maladaptive behaviours in therapy, patients learn to function in the world in such a way that they receive positive reinforcement. Several behaviour therapies devised to treat depression are characterized by overlapping behavioural and cognitive intervention strategies. These are:

(i) ***Self-Control Therapy:*** This therapy is developed by Lynn Rehm to treat depression. Key component of this approach include techniques designed to correct deficits in the patient's ability to realistically and productively self-monitor, self-evaluate and self-reinforce.

(ii) ***Social Learning Therapy:*** Peter Lewinsohn develops this therapy. The focus of this therapy is on increasing pleasant activities and interactions with the environments.

(iii) ***Social Skill Training:*** This approach is designed by Michel Hersen and Alan S. Bellack. It focuses on the training of social skills in parents to increase positive interactions and reinforcements.

The goal of behaviour therapies is to increase the frequency of the patient's positively reinforcing interactions with the environment and to decrease the number of negative interactions and also to improve social skills. Basically this therapy believes that alteration of personal behaviour is the most effective way to change the associated depressed thoughts and feelings.

(D) Family and Marital Therapy

Family therapy is not generally viewed as a primary therapy for the treatment of major depressive disorder, but increasing evidence indicates that helping a patient with a mood disorder reduce the chance of relapse. Family therapy examines the role the mood-disordered member in the overall psychological well being of the whole family; it also examines the role of the entire family in the maintenance of the patient's symptoms.

In addition, for married people who are depressed and having marital discord, it has been shown that marital therapy (focusing on the marital discord rather than depressed spouse alone) is as effective as cognitive therapy in reducing unipolar depression for the depressed spouse.

(E) Psychoanalytically Oriented Psychotherapy

All psychoanalytic contributions to studies of depression derive from the theory that a disturbance in interpersonal relations in early childhood, usually involving a loss or disappointment, impairs subsequent interpersonal relations. The affected person is especially vulnerable to interpersonal disappointments and loses later in life, which may result in depressive illness. The goal of traditional psychoanalytic psychotherapy is to elicit changes in personality structure, not simply to alleviate symptoms. It aims to improve the patient's potential for interpersonal trust, intimacy, and generativity; coping mechanisms, the ability to experience a wide range of emotions; and the capacity to grieve.

2

Literature Review, Objectives and Hypotheses

Literature review is an essential and very significant part of any research. It helps the researcher to conceptualize the problem in a better way by showing various perspectives of the problem. It provokes thinking on various aspects of the problem. Literature review also gives an idea to hypothesize the problem correctly.

In the present study the findings of previous researchers on various aspects of the depression were reviewed. For the convenience of the readers the literature review has been classified and presented under following broad heads:

- Symptoms of Depression.
- General Physical Health and Depression.
- Prevalence and Epidemiology of Depression.
- Psychosocial Characteristics of Depressed Patients.
- Adolescence and Depression.
- Old Age and Depression.
- Eating Habits of Depressed Patients.
- Addiction and Depression.
- Gender and Depression.
- Self and Depression.
- Interpersonal Relationship and Depression.
- Other Relevant Studies.

Symptoms of Depression

Brummet et al., (2000) sought to evaluate the associations between depressive symptoms and social support in a sample

of 115 depressed elderly patients using multi-measure approach to assess both depressive symptomatology and social support. They examined the baseline relations among a self-report measure of depressive symptoms, clinical assessments of depressive symptoms, and subjective and received social support, and also the ability of social support to predict changes in clinical assessments of depressive symptoms at 6 months and 1 year. The findings showed that baseline subjective support was negatively related to self-reports of depressive symptoms, but unrelated to clinical assessments at baseline or follow-up. Conversely, received support was unrelated to self-reported depressive symptoms, but positively related to both clinical assessments at baseline. However, higher ratings of received support at baseline predicted decreases in clinical ratings of depressive symptoms at 6 months and 1 year. These results have important implications for interpreting clinical data in elderly depressed patients. Specifically, when depressive symptoms are assessed using clinician ratings, the most informative aspect of social support with respect to future clinical status appears to be received, rather than perceived, support measures.

Psychosocial coping resources have been found to protect against depressive symptoms in people with and without chronic diseases. To estimate the direct and buffer effects of psychosocial resources on depression, and to examine whether these effects are different for various chronic diseases. Bisschop et al., (2004) conducted a longitudinal study covering 2288 community-dwelling respondents aged from 55-85 using structured interview method for assessing depressive symptoms, social support and personal coping resources, physical functioning and socio-demographic variables. Generalized estimating equation models were estimated for each disease, social support and personal coping resources. All resources, except social network size, showed a direct effect on depressive symptoms regardless of the presence of chronic diseases. Having a partner, high self-esteem, mastery, self-efficacy and feelingless lonely additionally buffered the negative effect of some, but not all, specific chronic diseases.

Unexpectedly, in patients with cardiac disease, none of the psychosocial resources exerted a buffer effect on depressive symptoms. For instrumental and emotional support only direct (unfavourable) effects and no buffer effects could be observed. Finally they concluded that buffer effects of psychosocial resources are different across various chronic diseases. This suggests that interventions to enhance specific resources may ameliorate depressive symptoms in specific chronic patients groups.

General Physical Health and Depression

Chronic Painful Physical Condition (CPPC) lasting 6 months or more influences the frequency and severity of depressive symptoms in subjects with Major Depressive Disorder (MDD). According to Ohayon (2004) CPPC is present in nearly half of subjects with MDD. CPPCs increase the severity of physical symptoms of depression (fatigue, insomnia nearly everyday, psychomotor retardation, weight gain). Moreover, CPPCs affect the duration of depressive episodes and their recurrence.

Sullivan et al., (2004) carried out a research on depression and health status among patients with coronary disease covering 113 outpatients with advanced heart failure of which 19.0% (n=21) had major depression or dysthymia, 9.0% (n=10) had minor depression, and 72.0% (n=82) had no current depression diagnosis. This study revealed that depressive group differed in severity of self-reported breathlessness, chest pain, and fatigue. Subject, and spouse-reported physical and role function also differed between the groups. Finally they concluded that depression is prospectively associated with poorer health status in patients with advanced heart failure. Physical and role function, symptom severity, and quality of life are all significantly affected.

The links between the psychological and physiological features of cancer risk and progression have been studied through psychoneuroimmunology. The persistent activation of the Hypothalamic-Pituitary-Adrenal (HPA) axis in the chronic stress response and in depression probably impairs the immune response and contributes to the development and progression of some types of cancer. The consecutive stages of the multi step immune reactions are either inhibited or enhanced as a result of previous or parallel stress experiences, depending on the type and intensity of the stressor and on the animal species, strain, sex, or age. In general, both stressors and depression are associated with the decreased cytotoxic T-cell and natural-killer-cell activities that affect processes such as immune surveillance of tumours, and with the events that modulate development and accumulation of somatic mutations and genomic instability (Reiche et al., 2004).

There is increasing evidence that major depression impacts the course of HIV infection to investigate predictors of depression (e.g., demographic and clinical variables, negative life events, and coping response) in people living with HIV/AIDS. Olley et.al., (2004) carried out a research among outpatients with recently diagnosed HIV/AIDS patients in South Africa. One hundred forty-nine recently diagnosed HIV/AIDS patients (44 males and 105 females) were evaluated. Subjects were assessed using the Mini International Neuropsychiatric Interview (MINI), the Carver Brief COPE coping scale, and the Sheehan Disability Scale. In addition, previous exposures to trauma and past risk behaviours were also assessed. Three variables gender, confidence interval, impact of negative life events, and disability predicted current major depression. It is well known from non-HIV populations that female gender and increased negative life events predict depression. These data also emphasize the importance of these links in HIV.

Depression is a significant psychiatric condition of childhood and adolescence. Again people with a chronic medical problem are at increased risk for developing depression. In this area Wray et al., (2004) conducted a research on 'Depression in pediatric patients before and 1 year after heart or heart-lung transplantation'. They administered the Mood and Feelings Questionnaire, a rating scale of depressive symptoms to 58 children before transplantation and to 46 children after transplantation. They found that children before transplantation suffer from more depression then children after transplantation. Transplantation is associated with a reduction in the prevalence of depressive symptomatology.

The study of Lichtenberger et al., (2003) examined the relationships between physiological function (i.e., both functional status and functional capacity), depressive symptoms, and body image among maintenance cardiac rehabilitation participants. In order to achieve their objective they studied 72 men (mean age = 67.3 years) all of whom had experienced a traumatic cardiac event (i.e., myocardial infraction, valve replacement surgery, coronary artery bypass graft surgery, percutaneous transluminal coronary angioplasty), and had completed some type of physician-supervised acute cardiac rehabilitation. Measures of body image (social physique, anxiety and body appearance satisfaction), self-reported functional status, clinician-reported functional capacity, and depressive symptoms were collected. The findings revealed that both functional capacity and functional status explained significant variance in social physique anxiety, whereas only functional status was a significant predictor of body appearance satisfaction. On the basis of the results they inferred that both patient perceptions of functional status and clinical measures of functional capacity are important aspects of psychosocial well-being among cardiac patients.

Hysterectomy is a surgical procedure that significantly affects the quality in which the operated person views herself, lowers self-esteem and brings about changes in the quality of life. The course of the post-operative period and the return of the patients to full health are largely affected by their psychological state and the quality of life they experience. A successful (in a medical sense) surgical procedure is not a guarantee of the bringing back health in a holistic sense. Many studies (Jawor et al., 2001) and clinical observations show that half of the group of women operated suffer from anxiety-depressive disorders as a cause of the operation, and a quarter of all those operated require specialist help. No psychological preparation for the operation, absence of closest people in the decision-making before the operation, lack of knowledge on the surgical operational-span, lacking psychological aid after the operation, all these can significantly affect the rehabilitation and the process of regaining the social functions. The appearance of depressive symptoms post-operatively as well as the earlier presence of affective disorder symptoms can be prognostic in the further development of the disorder. The early diagnosis of the affective disorder and the higher level of anxiety in women post-hysterectomy and the fast application of appropriate treatment can inhibit further symptom elevation and persistence.

Pincus et al., (1996) investigated the prevalence of self-reported depressive symptoms in a case-control study of patients with Rheumatoid Arthritis (RA) attending an outpatient clinic at the Middlesex Hospital. Patients selected their own controls, matched for age and sex. A total of 163 patients (77.0% of the sample) and 115 matched pairs completed the Hospital Anxiety and Depression Scale (HADS). The results indicated that RA patients are more depressed and anxious than controls. The prevalence of depression above the cut-point was 15 per cent.

Several factors have been related to depression for people with diabetes, but mechanisms of depression in this population remain unclear. In this regard Bailey et al., (1996) carried out a research to test mastery and self-esteem as mediators of disease-related depression in people with diabetes. A sample of 180 adults ages 21 to 81 were participated in this cross-sectional, co-relational study. Bailey et al., found that effect of diabetes on daily activities had a significant, direct (i.e., non-mediated) relationship to depressive symptoms. The entire model predicted 53.0% of variance in depression scores ($p = .0001$). These findings suggest nursing strategies for managing depression in patients with diabetes.

Depression is a common problem in patients with Parkinson's disease. It is thought that neuro-chemical changes contribute to its occurrence, but it is unclear why some patients develop depression and others do not. So Schrag et al., (2001) investigated the contributions of impairment, disability and handicap to depression in Parkinson's disease using a community-based sample of patients with Parkinson's disease. Research findings revealed that depression in patients with Parkinson's disease is associated with advancing disease severity, recent disease deterioration and occurrence of falls. Regression analysis suggests that depression in Parkinson's disease is more strongly influenced by the patients' perceptions of handicap than by actual disability. The treatment of depression should therefore be targeted independently of treatment of the motor symptoms of Parkinson's disease, and consider the patients' own perception of their disease.

Shnek et al., (2001) conducted a research on psychological factors and depressive symptoms in ischemic heart disease with the aim to determine whether learned helplessness, cognitive distortions, self-efficacy, and dispositional optimism assessed at Time 1 (T1; questionnaires mailed at 1 month post discharge) would predict depressive symptoms at Time 2 (T2; questionnaires mailed at 1-year follow-up) in a sample of 86 patients hospitalized with ischemic heart disease. Multiple regression results indicated that optimism and cognitive distortions at T1 were significantly associated with T1 depressive symptoms after controlling for confounding variables. When the T1 psychological factors were analyzed with T2 depressive symptoms, only optimism continued to predict depressive symptoms after controlling for confounds and T1 depressive symptoms.

Depression is associated with many physical problems. Wilson et al., (2002) conducted a prospective case-control study to determine whether patients with glaucoma have more depressive symptoms than patients without glaucoma. They administered the Center for Epidemiologic Studies Depression Scale (CES-D) and Composite International Diagnostic Interview, Short Form (CIDI-SF) questionnaires to all the study subjects to gather demographic information and medical history. The results showed that depression scores for patients with glaucoma do not differ significantly from scores of control patients. Having past or present mental illness is the only consistent predictor for depression in both the groups. Among glaucoma patients, visual acuity level, visual field severity, and use of topical beta-blockers are not predictors for depression. Finally on the basis they draw the conclusion that patients with glaucoma do not report being more depressed than patients without glaucoma as measured by the CES-D and the CIDI-SF questionnaires.

Stigmatization by the general population and their negative attitudes towards leprosy negatively impacts on patients' mental health, and so doe's patients' perception of that stigma too. Tsutsumi et al., (2004) conducted a study with the view to assess the depressive status of leprosy patients, the patient perception of that stigma, and its association with their depressive status in Dhaka, Bangladesh covering 140 patients, and a selected comparison group of 135 local people without any chronic diseases using Centre for Epidemiologic Studies Depression Scale (CES-D) Bengali version. The findings of the study revealed that the depressive status in leprosy patients is greater than that of the general public. Further, actual experiences of discrimination are based on the stigma associated with the depressive status of leprosy patients. Tsutsumi et al., suggested that mental health care for patients, regulation of discriminatory action and education is important to decrease the social stigma among the general population about leprosy, for improving the mental health of Bangladeshi leprosy patients.

Silverstone et al., (1996) carried out a study covering 186 patients in a view to determining the prevalence of major depressive disorder in acutely ill medical inpatients, and the relationship of this to low self-esteem. The results showed that 18 patients (9.7%) were depressed. The depressed patients were significantly younger than the non-depressed patients and were significantly more likely to be female. The depressed patients had a significantly lower self-esteem than the non-depressed patients, whose self-esteem was no different from the general population. However, the depressed patients were not more severely ill than the non-depressed patients. The results also demonstrated that both nurses and physicians were poor at recognizing the presence of major depression. The findings also revealed that the prevalence rates for MDD in medical patients is between 5.0% to 10.0% rather than the previously accepted range of 20.0% to 40.0%.

Prevalence and Epidemiology of Depression

Epidemiological studies in western societies generally show that depressive episodes occur in 10.0-20.0% of pregnant women. Longitudinal studies have demonstrated that antenatal depression is one of the most powerful predictors of postnatal depression. There is also a growing literature that shows that antenatal psychological distress can adversely affect maternal health and well-being.

Lee et al., (2004) carried out a study on antenatal depression among 238 pregnant Chinese women (38 weeks of pregnancy) and found that a significant proportion of Chinese women suffer from psychiatric morbidity during pregnancy. Depressive disorders are by far the commonest morbidity in the study population. Given the scope of the morbidity and the potential impact on obstetric and neonatal outcomes, early screening and treatment are warranted.

O'Sullivan (2004) conducted a cross-sectional study on the psychosocial profile of patients with depressive patients comparing depressive risk factors within and between two Western community cohorts covering six hundred eight primary care patients from the rural population of Farranfore, Ireland, and the suburban population of Penrith, Australia. The survey included the Centre for Epidemiological Study Depression Scale, Vulnerable Personality Style Questionnaire, Life Events Inventory, and Social Support Survey. Exposure to a range of early adverse childhood events was also assessed. The three month prevalence of depressive symptoms between Farranfore and Penrith respondents were 30.0% and 35.0%, respectively. O'Sullivan (2004) observed that the onset of depressive symptoms was positively associated with unfavourable childhood events, poorly perceived social supports, recent stressful life events, a vulnerable personality style, and previous depressive illness. The study identifies the person's social and internal world as a potent source of depressive risk over the lifespan.

Psychosocial Characteristics of Depressed Patients

In depressive disorders, there are psychopathological dimensions other than depressed mood and anxiety that deserve greater clinical recognition and research. Pasquini et al., (2004) attempted a research to assess the relevance of anger, irritability, aggressiveness, hostility, and psychomotor activation in major depressive disorder. A total of 222 newly admitted consecutive outpatients with major depressive disorder (mean age 48.9 years, 64.4% females) were enrolled in the study. They obtained a three-factor solution accounting for 47.4% of total variance. The factors were interpreted as 'anger/irritability', 'depression', and 'anxiety', respectively. The anger/irritability dimension was clinically relevant in 23.0% of patients. Anger/aggressiveness was especially frequent (21.6%), whereas psychomotor activation was infrequent (0.9%). Finally their study suggests that one of these symptom clusters (i.e. depressed mood and anxiety) includes anger, irritability, aggressiveness, and hostility.

Bienvenu et al., in the year 2004 observed that all of the lifetime disorders of interest (simple phobia, social phobia, agoraphobia, panic disorder, Obsessive-Compulsive Disorder (OCD), Generalized Anxiety Disorder, Major Depressive Disorder (MDD), and Dysthymia were associated with high neuroticism. Social phobia, agoraphobia, and dysthymia were associated with low extraversion, and OCD was associated with high openness to experience.

In addition, they also found that lower-order factors of extraversion (E), openness (O), agreeableness (A), and conscientiousness (C) were associated with certain disorders (specifically, low assertiveness (E) and high openness to feelings (O) with MDD, low trust (A) with social phobia and agoraphobia, low self-discipline (C) with several of the disorders, and low competence and achievement striving (C) with social phobia. Neuroticism in particular was related to acuity of disorder.

Gunderson et al., (2004) investigate the longitudinal association of changes in Major Depressive Disorder (MDD) and borderline personality disorder among a sample of 161 patients with borderline personality disorder who have been followed with repeated measures at 6, 12, 24, and 36 months are investigated to see whether those with co-occurring MDD differ at baseline and in their course. Proportional hazard regression and cross-lagged panel analyses are used to demonstrate whether changes in the course of either disorder have predictable effects on the course of the other. They found that when borderline personality disorder and MDD co-occur, they can sometimes have independent courses, but more often improvements in MDD are predicted by prior improvements in borderline personality disorder. Their findings suggested that clinicians should not ignore borderline personality disorder in hopes that treatment of MDD will be followed by improvement of borderline personality disorder.

Depression is common among adolescents, and suicide is the third leading cause of death among 15 to 19 years old. Hallfors et al., (2004) conducted a research on adolescent depression and suicide risk association with sex and drug behaviour. They studied the relationship among the health problems, which are associated with drug use and early sexual intercourse. They found that young individuals who abstain from risk behaviours; involvement in any drinking, smoking, and/or sexual activity is associated with significantly increased odds of depression, suicidal ideation, and suicide attempts. Odds ratios are highest among youth who engaged in illegal drug use. There are few differences between boys and girls who abstain from sex and drug behaviours. Girls are less likely than boys to engage in high-risk behaviours, but those who did tended to be more vulnerable to depression, suicidal ideation, and suicide attempt. Finally they concluded that teens engaging in risk behaviours are at increased odds for depression, suicidal ideation, and suicide attempts.

Clinical depression and other psychological disorders are associated with suicidal ideation, attempts, and deaths. Because of the link between suicide and mental illness, whenever discussion of "assisted suicide" arises, the possibility that major depression is affecting the decision arises. Werth et al., (2004) found that clinical depression is closely related to suicide, "assisted suicide," and other decisions that will hasten death (i.e. withholding and withdrawing treatment, terminal sedation, and voluntarily stopping eating and drinking).

According to Phillips et al., (2004) patients with both depression and drug dependence are at an elevated risk for suicide, yet suicide remains rare and difficult to predict. Female gender, violent behaviour in the past thirty days and lifetime, and less education are correlated with a history of suicide attempts. Family conflict and depression severity is also correlated with current suicidal ideation.

Kuo et al., (2004) attempted a research with an aim to examine if hopelessness is a long-term predictor of suicidal behaviours using a longitudinal study design with a community sample of more than 3,000 participants. They assessed the association of hopelessness at baseline and incident of suicidal behaviours in the 13-years follow-up period, adjusting for the presence of depression and substance use disorders. Suicide behaviours studied included completed suicide, self-reported attempted suicide, and suicide ideation. They found that hopelessness is predictive of all three types of suicidal behaviours in the follow-up period, even after adjustment. The association between suicidality and hopelessness is stronger and more stable than the association of suicidality with the presence of depression and substance use disorders. Finally they concluded that hopelessness is an independent risk factor for completed suicide, suicide attempts, and suicidal ideation.

Traumatic Brain Injury (TBI) is associated with psychiatric illness, suicidal ideation, suicide attempts, and completed suicide. Oquendo et al., (2004) investigated the relationship between mild TBI and other risk factors for suicidal behaviour in major depressive episode. They hypothesized that mild TBI would be associated with suicidal behaviour at least partly because of shared risk factors that contribute to the diathesis for suicidal acts. Depressed patients (N = 325) presenting for treatment were evaluated for psychopathology, traumatic history, and suicidal behaviour. Data were analyzed using Student t-test, chi-square statistic, or Fisher exact test. A backward step-wise logistic regression model (N=255) examined the relationship between attempter status and variables that differed in the TBI and non-TBI patients. Forty-four per cent of all subjects reported mild TBI. Subjects with TBI were more likely to be male, have a history of substance abuse, have cluster B personality disorder, and be more aggressive and hostile compared with subjects without TBI. They were also more likely to be suicide attempters, although their suicidal behaviour was not different from that of suicide attempters without TBI. Attempt status was mostly predicted by aggression and hostility, but not the presence of TBI. For males, a history of TBI increased the likelihood of being a suicide attempter, whereas the risk was elevated for females regardless of TBI history.

Self-criticism is a unique personality dimension in different forms of psychopathology including depression. (Blatt, 1991). The study of Cox et al., (2000) revealed that depressive patients scored significantly higher on self-criticism dimension measured by the Depressive Experiences Questionnaire (DEQ).

Personality traits confer risk for suicidal behaviours in middle age and older adults. Useda et al., (2004) examined the contribution of personality traits to attempted suicide, the number of suicidal attempts, and suicidal ideation in a sample of depressed inpatients. They assessed personality using the Revised NEO Personality Inventory (NEO-PI-R). Bivariate analyses showed that suicide attempters were more self-conscious, self-effacing, impulsive, and vulnerable to stress, and less warm, gregarious, and inclined to experience positive emotions. Multivariate regression analyses controlling for age, gender, severity of depression, and psychiatric comorbidity showed that patients with a lifetime history of attempted suicide were less inclined to experience positive emotions and be more self-effacing. Patients with more severe suicidal ideation were less warm and more self-effacing.

Adolescence and Depression

To verify the hypothesis that family stress variables are associated with the effects of maternal depression on offspring diagnoses and also to examine whether such factors may be differentially associated with disorders in offspring of depressed and never-depressed women, Hammen et al., (2004) conducted a study on eight hundred sixteen (816) mothers and their 15-year-old children in an Australian community. Significant interaction effects were found between maternal depression and family discord/stress variables such that high levels of environmental risk factors were significantly associated with youth depression in children of depressed women compared with low levels of adverse conditions and were generally less associated with depression in children of non-depressed women. Non-depressive disorders were associated with adverse family and stress factors for both groups of children. The results suggest that psychosocial factors may contribute to diagnoses in offspring of depressed women in community samples.

Starling et al., (2004) examined changes in prevalence of psychological disturbance over time in adolescents referred for treatment. They measured the type and severity of emotional and behavioural problems using the Youth Self-Report and Child Behaviour Checklist in 4495 clinic-referred adolescents aged 12-17 years, born in a 21-year period (1966-1986). The findings revealed that there are significant increases in reports of self-harm and suicidal ideation (5.0% and 4.0% increase in odds per year, respectively) according to the parents of the referred adolescence. In contrast, there are no changes over time in the adolescents' reports. Neither parents nor children reported an increase in depressive symptoms. Finally they concluded that perceptions of a secular increase might reflect increasing parental awareness of some behaviour, particularly self-harm and suicidal ideation.

Otsuki et al., (2003) tested the relationship of self-esteem and depression with alcohol, tobacco, and other drug (ATOD) use in a California statewide sample of more than 4,300 Asian

American high school students comprising five sub-groups: Chinese, Japanese, Korean, Filipino, and Vietnamese. Estimated prevalence rates of alcohol, tobacco, and marijuana use among males and females from these Asian American subgroups are presented. Correlations revealed that cigarette, alcohol, and marijuana use were generally more related to high depression and low self-esteem in females than in males. The results of the study indicated that for females, depression was significantly related to alcohol and tobacco use, but self-esteem was not. Neither self-esteem nor depression was a significant contributor to marijuana use.

The survey of Angold and Costello (1993) on depression revealed important difference between preadolescents and adolescent groups. Their findings revealed that depression is fairly rare—affecting 2% to 3% of the youngsters who are below age 12. On the other hand adolescents have higher rates (6.0-8.0%).

Adult-onset cases of DSM-III-R Major Depressive Disorder (MDD) often have had a history of mood disturbances and allied clinical features during childhood or adolescence. The study of Wilcox et al., (2004) seeks to illuminate these early-life disturbances, as recalled and reported by adult-onset MDD cases (i.e. those whose first episode of MDD occurred after age 18) and non-cases covering 1920 patients. Of the 1920 participants, 150 were found to have a history of adult-onset MDD; 1755 were sub-threshold with respect to DSM criteria or reported few or no depression-related problems. Survival analysis was used to plot and study the cumulative occurrence of each clinical feature of depression from age 6 through 18 years for cases of adult-onset MDD versus non-cases. Results indicated that the earliest and most frequently occurring forerunners of adult-onset MDD were persistent depressed mood, anhedonia, feelings of worthlessness, and thoughts of death or suicide, with persistent anhedonia and worthlessness having a special prognostic value. One-third of adult-onset cases of MDD reported at least one clinical feature before age 19 versus only 7.3% of non-cases.

Associations between parenting style and depressive symptomatology in a community sample of young adolescents

(N = 2596) were investigated by Martin et al., (2004). They used self-report measures including the Parental Bonding Instrument and the Center for Epidemiological Studies Depression Scale. They compared the 25-item 2-factor and 3-factor models by Parker et al. (1979), Kendler et al., (1996) 16-item 3-factor model, and Parker et al., (1983) quadrant model for the Parental Bonding Instrument. Data analysis included analysis of variance and logistic regression. Reanalysis of Parker et al., original scale indicates that overprotection is composed of separate factors: intrusiveness (at the individual level) and restrictiveness (in the social context). All models reveal significant independent contributions from paternal care, maternal care, and maternal overprotection (2-factor) or intrusiveness (3-factor) to moderate and serious depressive symptomatology, controlling for sex and family living arrangement. Additive rather than multiplicative interactions between care and overprotection were found. Finally they concluded that regardless of the level of parental care and affection, clinicians should note that maternal intrusiveness is strongly associated with adverse psychosocial health in young adolescents.

Old Age and Depression

The article of O' Connor et al., (2001) examined some of the factors responsible for older patients' decision to report current depressive symptoms to their general medical practitioner. They conducted this survey on a stratified sample of 1,021 patients aged 70+ years of 30 GPs in Melbourne, Australia, to measure the prevalence of depressive symptoms, the frequency with which patients had informed GPs of their symptoms, and GPs' recognition of major depressive episodes. Patients and informants were questioned using the Canberra Interview for the Elderly, which generates rigorous ICD-10 research diagnoses. Logistic regression analysis showed that symptom disclosure was associated in descending order of importance with higher depressive scores, previous contact with a psychiatrist, and female gender. Even so, 48.0% of persons with

ICD-10 moderate or severe depressive episode had not reported any current complaints to their doctor at the time of interview. Finally they inferred that older patients often do not report depressive symptoms to their medical practitioner. Men and patients lacking 'psychological mindedness' may be at special risk.

A number of studies have concluded that the perceived quality of support is more strongly associated with mental health than with the actual structure of personal networks. The study of Lynch et al., (1999) examined clinical, historical, and phenomenological variables associated cross-sectionally and longitudinally with perceived social support. Participants included elderly, middle-aged, and young-adult depressed samples were derived from the Duke Clinical Research Centre for the Study of Depression in Late Life. Cross-sectional multivariate analyses revealed that perceived social support was: (1) for the elderly associated with pessimistic thinking, being divorced, having strange ideas, the degree of social interaction, and instrumental support; (2) for middle-age associated with dysthymia, divorce, pessimistic thoughts, social interaction, and instrumental support; and (3) among young adults with instrumental support only. Longitudinal multivariate analyses indicated that only perceived social support at Time 1 predicted perceived social support 1 year later among elderly and middle-aged subjects, whereas only instrumental support predicted perceived social support 1 year later among the young-adult sample. The findings of this study indicate that in addition to whatever else clinicians do for depressed patients, they must endeavour to address relationship or social support difficulties, especially in the elderly.

Post-Traumatic Stress Disorder (PTSD) and major depression are frequently comorbid. Age and major depression are associated with higher cortisol levels and dexamethasone resistance, whereas PTSD is associated with lower cortisol and dexamethasone supersensitivity. Some researchers found that Cortisol levels increase with age in depressed patients without PTSD but not in depressed patients with PTSD or in healthy volunteers (Sher et al., 2004). The study of Sher et al., highlighted the importance of considering age in psychobiology.

Wallace and O'Hara (1992) studied changes in depressive symptoms in a rural sample of people aged 65 and over. They found significant increases overtime in depressive symptoms—especially among the very old, age 85 and above—suggesting that late life may be a time of increased depression risk.

Eating Habits of Depressed Patients

Fava et al., (1997) carried out a study on one hundred thirty-nine outpatients (82 women and 57 men) with Major Depressive Disorder (MDD) in a view to evaluate the relationship between eating disorder symptomatology and severity of depression in depressed outpatients before and after anti-depressant treatment and also to assess the effect of treatment on eating disorder symptomatology. On the basis of the study findings Fava et al., suggest that several symptoms characteristic of eating disordered patients are linked to the severity of depressive symptoms. Decreases in eating disorder symptomatology following anti-depressant treatment may be related to changes in depressive symptoms.

Both depressive disorders and eating disorders are multi-dimensional and heterogeneous disorders. The paper of Casper et al., (1998) examines the nature of their relationship by reviewing clinical descriptive, family-genetic, treatment, and biological studies that relate to the issue. The studies confirm the prominence of depressive symptoms and depressive disorders in eating disorders. Other psychiatric syndromes, which occur with less frequency, such as anxiety disorders and obsessive-compulsive disorders in anorexia nervosa, or personality disorders, anxiety disorders, and substance abuse in bulimia nervosa, also play an important role in the development and maintenance of eating disorders.

Diet may affect mood and cognitive functions. But Hakkarainen et al., (2003) found no consistent association between dietary intake of amino acids and low mood or depressed mood and risk of suicide.

Addiction and Depression

Depression and co-morbid substance abuse disorders are a major public health problem. Again depression among patients with substance abuse problems is a common problem. In this regard Manwell et al., conducted a study in the year 2004 on 30-days and lifetime prevalence of major depression among heavy drinking population (227) selected from 12 Polish primary care clinics. They defined heavy drinking as more than 20 drinks per week for males, or more than 13 drinks per week for females, or consumption of more than four drinks five or more times in the previous 30 days, or two or more positive replies to the CAGE questions. Criteria from the Diagnostic and Statistical Manual were used to assess lifetime and past 30-days depression. Results showed that 35.0% of women and men met criteria for depression in the 30-days prior to the interview. Lifetime rates were 45.0% for women and 52.0% for men. Men and women with a CAGE score of 4 were at higher risk for both 30-days (67.0%) and lifetime (78.0%) depression. Recreational drug users and patients reporting symptoms of anti-social personality disorders were at increased risk for lifetime depression. Subjects reporting symptoms of a childhood conduct disorder were at higher risk for 30-day depression.

Many researches have highlighted the relationship between cigarette smoking and depressive symptoms. Again in the year 2004, Brook et al., examined the relationship between cigarette smoking and depressive symptoms in a longitudinal sample of 688 adolescents and young adults through surveys conducted over 13 years. The results of their study indicate that a history of earlier cigarette smoking in adolescence predicts later depressive symptoms in the late twenties. The study also suggests that depressive symptoms during adolescence predict cigarette smoking in the late twenties but not above and beyond prior smoking. These results help to clarify and expand current knowledge on the links between cigarette smoking and depression and also focus on several clinical implications for treatment of both cigarette smoking and depressive symptoms among both adolescents and young adults.

Friedman et al., (2004) conducted a research on depression, negative self-image, and suicidal attempts as effects of substance use and substance dependence. The main purpose of their study was to compare, separately by gender, the degree to which cocaine use/abuse, marijuana use/abuse, and alcohol use/abuse each predict to developing either: a state of depression, or a negative self-image, or a negative personal outlook or for making a suicidal attempt covering 431 subjects, at average age of 37. They found that female alcoholics and drug addicts have strong negative self-image as well as negative personal outlook, while males are relatively more predicted to making suicide attempts. Of the three types of substances, cocaine use/abuse predicted to the greatest number of negative outcomes; and alcohol use/abuse predicted to no negative outcomes.

Many psychiatric interviews with opiate addicts are characterized by three features: (1) the patient has a very factual and objective conversation, (2) the evaluation of the autobiographical memory is very difficult, (3) there is a high prevalence of affective disorders responsible for an impairment in cognitive functions.

Eiber et al., (1999) conducted a research on a group of opiate addicts with the aim to estimate the impact of depression on the ability to produce autobiographical recollection in a population of opiate addicts and also to compare episodic and semantic autobiographical memory among opiate addicts and healthy controls. Participants were consecutive attendees of a methadone outpatient clinic who are multiple drug dependent patients consuming mainly heroine. The first investigation took place in entry and after two months. Eiber et al., selected 21 patients with a mean duration of intoxication of 11 years. Ten of these patients have been investigated again after 2 months and 8 of them have been included in a methadone maintenance programme. The patients' investigation comprised two parts: first, the evaluation of autobiographical memory (only assessed at entry of the study) with an autobiographical fluency test and the semi-structured autobiographical memory interview of Kopelman; second, the psychiatric assessment included self-rating questionnaires and observer-rating questionnaires. They noticed that opiate addicts showed a decrease in episodic autobiographical memory but an increase in semantic affective memory and objective modalization. In the fluency test, there was no difference in the number of evoked items between opiate addicts and healthy controls. This study suggests the implication of the drugs in the emergence of memory deficits. The improvement of depressive symptomatology after two months occurring without psychotropic drugs suggests the transient feature of depression and emphasises on non-pharmacological aspects of treatment.

Cornelius et al., (1995) made an attempt to provide a comprehensive description of the clinical features of patients who presented to an intake psychiatric setting with major depression and alcohol dependence and to determine which clinical features distinguished this dual-diagnosis group from patients with the two relevant single diagnoses. The findings revealed that the psychiatric symptom that most strongly distinguished the depressed alcoholics from the two comparison groups was the level of suicidal. The depressed alcoholics differed significantly from the non alcoholic depressed patients on only two depressive symptoms, suicidality (59.0% higher) and low self-esteem (22.0% higher); they were also significantly distinguished from the non-alcoholic depressed patients by factors such as greater impulsivity, functional impairment, and abnormal personal and social history markers

Gender and Depression

Williams et al., (1995) carried out a study on gender differences in the frequency and manifestation of depression in primary care. They found that more women than men were diagnosed as having a mood disorder (31.0 vs. 19.0; $p < 0.01$), and an anti-depressant was newly prescribed only for women ($p < 0.001$). There were no gender differences in physician ratings of patients' health, but women rated their health significantly more poorly than did men.

Similarly, functional impairment scores were significantly lower in women than in men. Finally they concluded that women are much more likely than men to have depressive disorders, and when these disorders are diagnosed, to receive a prescription for anti-depressant medication.

Studies investigating the correlates of adolescent depression and suicidal tendencies have found that the probability of such tendencies vary from race to race and from gender to gender. Sen (2004) conducted a research on 'Adolescent Propensity for Depressed Mood and Help Seeking: Race and Gender Differences' with the aim to test whether there are significant differences between genders, and between non-Hispanic whites, non-Hispanic blacks, Hispanics and Asians in the likelihood of seeking help, and from whom, when depressed on a sample of more than 9000 adolescents enrolled in grades 6-10. He used Multinomial logit models to estimate the likelihood of being depressed or at self-injury risk, and help-seeking behaviour in event of depressed mood. Models are estimated for the full sample and sub-samples who report depressed mood or are at self-injury risk. In addition to race and gender, all models control for additional demographic characteristics such as age, family structure, and family socio-economic status. Results showed that adolescent females are significantly more likely than adolescent males to suffer from depressed mood. However, adolescent males are less likely to ask for help than females (odds ratio: 0.72). All minority groups are more likely to suffer from depressed mood compared to non-Hispanic whites, but blacks are at lower self-injury risk. Blacks and Asians are especially prone not to ask for help, with the problem being particularly acute in case of black males and Asian males.

Prochazka and Agren (2003) carried out research on aggression and cerebral monoaminergic turnover covering sixty-six patients (40 women and 26 men) with Persistent Depressive Disorder (PDD). The study subjects were compared with 497 control subjects from the general Swedish population using the Aggression Questionnaire—Revised Swedish Version (AQ-RSV) to patients and control subjects. They found PDD patients more hostile than the general population. The results also suggest a clinically meaningful sex difference in a positive relationship between hostility and serotonergic/noradrenergic turnover in PDD patients.

Depression is associated with significant impairment and physical conditions and , thus, clearly constitutes a significant public health problem. 10 to 25 per cent of patients seen by primary care providers have some type of depressive disorder that affects not only their functioning and well-being, but also their physical health. The emergence of sex differences at puberty has generated a great deal of research into the biological (in particular, reproductive hormones) and psychosocial factors that may account for this difference and contribute to depression in women across the life cycle. The lifetime prevalence of major depression in women ranges from 10.0 to 23.0%, twice the rate among men; until puberty, however, rates are similar among boys and girls (Bromberger 2004).

Self and Depression

Bookless et al., (2002) conducted a prospective study on personal appraisal of the experience of a depressive disorder covering 61 patients suffering from depressive disorder who are receiving treatment for Major Depression using the Personal Appraisal Inventory (PAI) (Bookless, Clayer and McFarlane, 2000). They examined the subjects over a period of 7 months. They also examined the initial (Time 1) association between the individual items of the PAI and self-reported levels of depression, anxiety, disability, self-esteem and psychological distress. They found that these variables related to some items pertaining to appraisal of the harm and threat engendered by the disorder, but did not relate to appraisal of the positive and negative options for managing the disorder. Seven months later (Time 2) few significant changes were found in the way people appraised the impact of the disorder however, levels of depression, anxiety, disability and distress at Time 2 were predicted by several appraisal items.

Erectile dysfunction always has a psychological component in addition to the underlying physical cause. The extent of depression and reduced self-esteem in patients who present with erectile dysfunction are explored by Intili et al., (1998).

Dependency and self-criticism reflect relatively stable personality dimensions in patients with a mood disorder. According to Rosenfarb et al., (1998) dependency needs in depressed women are heavily influenced by mood state. Women with bipolar disorder in remission report fewer dependency needs than women with no history of psychiatric disorder. On the other hand self-criticism appears to be a characterological trait in both major depression and bipolar disorder.

De Bonis et al., (1998) made a comparative study to investigate the relationship between depressed mood and Borderline Personality Disorder (BPD) on self and others descriptions, with a special emphasis on the self-structure's valence, that is, its affective, negative and/or positive content covering seventeen unipolar depressed patients with associated BPD and twelve unipolar depressed patients without BPD. Further they compared this experimental group to a group of eighteen non-psychiatric controls on four measures of evaluation and of affective discrepancy of descriptions of self and others. The analysis of the findings showed that depressed patients with and without BPD differed from the non-psychiatric controls with regard to negativity of the descriptions. As compared with the two other groups, depressed patients with BPD showed a distinctive pattern characterized by the joint presence of a negative view of self and a larger affective discrepancy for others, with others being conjunctively assigned positive and negative attributes.

Young women seen in public care gynecology clinics are at very high risk for depression. In this regard Alvidrez et al., (1999) conducted a study to examine the rates and predictors of self-recognition of depression in a sample of 95 depressed public care women's clinic patients. They found that fewer than half of the women (44.0%) identified their problems as depression, but majority of them were not likely to receive treatment for their problems. Predictors of self-recognition included being told by a doctor in the past that they were depressed, endorsing medical/psychiatric causes of mental illness, and use of the coping strategies of facing a problem, alcohol or drug use, and prayer. These findings indicate the need for gynecology settings to: (1) provide education about depression to women, (2) encourage them to discuss emotional problems with their physicians, and (3) provide increased education and training to physicians and staff about depression detection and assessment.

Mood disorders are characterized by manic and depressive episodes alternating with normal mood. Serretti et al., (1999) attempted a research to focus on self-esteem and social adjustment in remitted mood disorders patients comparing patients with mood disorders (99 bipolar and 86 major depressive subjects, in remission) with a group of 100 control subjects using the self-esteem scale (SES) and the social adjustment scale (SAS) to measure self-esteem and social adjustment, respectively, in both groups of subjects. The results showed that patients with mood disorder exhibited worse social adjustment and lower self-esteem than control subjects, which again strongly confirm the previous findings that social functions are heavily impaired among patients with mood disorders.

Sheppard et al., (1996) examined the alternative explanations for the changes in thinking associated with depression. According to them depressive thinking could reflect a generalized increase in accessibility of negative constructs and memories, previously associated with depression. Alternatively, depressive thinking could reflect changes at a more generic level of cognitive representation, related to schematic mental models. To investigate contrasting predictions from these two explanations, depressed patients and non-depressed controls completed sentence stems involving social approval or personal achievement e.g. 'If I could always be right then others would-be'. Construct accessibility views predict that depression will be associated with more negative completions (e.g. 'dislike'). By contrast, the schematic model view predicts patients may give more positive completions (e.g. 'like'). This is because schematic models reflect inter-relationships between constructs, and, it is suggested, depression is associated with use of schematic mental models that imply closer dependence of personal worth/ acceptance on success/approval than the models used in the non-depressed state. The results suggest that depressive thinking reflects changes in the high level mental models used to interpret experience.

Hayward et al., (2002) conducted an exploratory study on Stigma and self-esteem in patients with manic depression. This study suggests a relationship between mood and self-esteem, while feelings of stigmatisation seem to be relatively independent of mood.

Studies of rumination suggest that self-focused attention is maladaptive and perpetuates depression. Conversely, self-focused attention can be adaptive, facilitating self-knowledge and the development of the alternative functional interpretations of negative thoughts and feelings on which cognitive therapy of depression depends. Increasing evidence suggests there are distinct varieties of self-focus, each with distinct functional properties. The study of Watkins et al., (2004) supports the differentiation of self-focus into distinct modes of self-attention with distinct functional effects in depression. They also support the usefulness of training recovered depressed patients in adaptive experiential forms of self-awareness, as in mindfulness-based cognitive therapy.

Interpersonal Relationship and Depression

Stern et al., (1997) carried out a study on interpersonal perceptions among patients with Borderline Personality Disorder (BPD). The objective of their study was to investigate the validity of object relation's theories. They compared depressed patients with BPD to patients with Major Depressive Disorder (MD) without BPD. Subjects were 77 male and female inpatients (BPD = 55, MD = 22). The mean ages were 30.5 for BPD subjects and 36.3 for MD subjects. Results showed consistency with the object relation's theory. Findings also revealed that BPD patients saw themselves as hostile, labile, and unstable where as MD patients avoid acknowledging and responding to relatives criticality.

Lam et al., (2003) postulated that depressed patients who engaged in self-focused rumination on their depressive symptoms may experience more hopelessness, more interpersonal distress and poorer social functioning while patients who distract themselves may experience less severe hopelessness and better social functioning. They selected one-hundred and nine (109) outpatients suffering from Major Depressive Disorders to understand their response style to depression, hopelessness and interpersonal style and also their levels of social functioning. Lam et al., found that rumination was associated with higher levels of depression and distraction was associated with lower levels of depression. Furthermore when levels of depression and gender were controlled for, rumination contributed to higher levels of hopelessness and distraction contributed to lower levels of hopelessness. Both rumination and levels of depression contributed significantly to higher levels of interpersonal distress when gender was controlled for. Ruminators were rated to have significantly more severe problems in intimate relationships while distracters were rated to have significantly higher social functioning.

Other Relevant Studies

Marmorstein et al., (2004) conducted a community based study on twins and their parents in a view to explore whether major depression and/or anti-social behaviour tended to occur more frequently among partners of depressed mothers (compared to partners of non-depressed mothers) and to examine how these paternal disorders related to offspring psychopathology. They interviewed depressed and non-depressed mothers, their partners (the biological fathers of the twins), and their 17-years-old offspring. The results showed that depressed mothers are tended to partner with anti-social fathers. Depression in mother and anti-social behaviour in father are both significantly and independently associated with offspring depression and conduct disorder.

Abi Daoud et al., (2004) examined depression, self-esteem, and mastery in the family caretakers of a group of males with Duchenne muscular dystrophy in comparison to a control group. A questionnaire based on the National Population Health Survey from Statistics Canada, a survey to collect information on the health of the Canadian population and related socio-demographic information, was conducted by telephone with 42 parents. The results were compared with the national data from the National Population Health Survey (1994 and 1999), matched for province of residence, number of children in the household, age, and marital status of the respondents. Parents of children with Duchenne muscular dystrophy had a higher probability of going through a major depressive episode and had significantly lower self-esteem and mastery scores than the national control group. Parents without a partner had lower scores on the mastery scale, and parents of males older than 13 years of age were more likely to experience distress that interfered with life.

Major depressive disorder is the most frequent comorbid condition in Obsessive-Compulsive Disorder (OCD). The study of Hong et al., (2004) investigated factors associated with the development of Recurrent Major Depressive Disorder (RDD) in patients with OCD covering 80 OCD cases and 73 control subjects. Two experienced psychiatrists independently reviewed all clinical materials and made final consensus diagnoses using DSM-IV criteria. Family history of OCD and RDD, additional comorbid disorders, OCD symptoms and illness severity were compared between persons with OCD alone (n = 21) and OCD with RDD (n = 41). Compared to OCD probands without RDD, OCD probands with RDD had earlier age at first diagnosis, more severe obsessive-compulsive symptoms, and were more likely to have a family history of RDD. Social Phobia, Separation Anxiety Disorder, and Body

Dimorphic Disorder occurred more frequently in the comorbid group. In a multiple logistic regression model, only early age of OCD diagnosis was significantly associated with RDD. Early age at onset of OCD increases the risk of depressive disorder in individuals with OCD.

Lobentanz et al., (2004) conducted a study in a series of 504 patients with Multiple Sclerosis (MS), to asses their quality of life, disability, depressive mood, fatigue severity and sleep quality in comparison with healthy individuals using Quality of Life Index, Expanded Disability Status Scale, Self-rating Depression Scale, Fatigue Severity Scale, and Pittsburgh Sleep Quality Index. They found that most patients were severely disabled; almost half were mildly to severely depressed, suffering from reduced sleep quality and/or fatigue. The multiple sclerosis patients had significantly lower quality of life. Finally they concluded that depressive mood is the main factor influencing QOL. The disability status, fatigue and reduced sleep quality have an impact mainly on physical domains of life quality.

The Beck Depression Inventory (BDI) is the most often used self-rating instrument for depressive symptoms. The study of Svanborg et al., (2001) compared the Beck Depression Inventory with a self-rating version of the Montgomery Asberg Depression Rating Scale (MADRS-S) among 86 psychiatric patients with mainly affective and anxiety disorders. They found that both the instruments were about equal in differentiating between different Axis-I diagnoses and did not differ according to sensitivity to change during anti-depressive treatment. Although the scales were highly intercorrelated (r = 0.869), the BDI was demonstrated to tap more maladaptive personality traits compared to the MADRS-S. Finally Svanborg et.al. concluded that the MADRS-S is equivalent to the BDI as a self-assessment instrument for depression, but the MADRSS focuses on core depressive symptoms, and is less influenced by maladaptive personality traits.

According to Iqbal et al., (2000) session in the acute stage remitted in line with the psychosis and that 36.0% of patients developed Post-Psychotic Depression (PPD). Again in the year

2000 Iqbal et al., apply their cognitive framework to PPD and chart the appraisal of self and psychosis and their link with the later emergence of PPD covering 105 Schizophrenic patients, who were followed up over 12 months following the acute episode, taking measures of depression, working self-concept, cognitive vulnerability, insight and appraisals of psychosis. Results of this study showed that before developing PPD, these patients felt greater loss, humiliation and entrapment by their illness than those who relapsed or did not become depressed, and were more likely to see their future selves in 'lower status' roles. Upon becoming depressed, participants developed greater insight, lower self-esteem and a worsening of their appraisals of psychosis. Finally they inferred that depression in psychosis arises from the individual's appraisal of psychosis and its implications for his/her perceived social identity, position and 'group fit'. Patients developing PPD feel forced to accept a subordinate role without opportunity for escape.

Bodlund (2000) stated that about 15.0% of primary care attendents suffer from depression, yet only a minority are identified and treated. It is of major importance to spread knowledge of the prevalence of depression and tools for recognizing the disorder. Most patients can be successfully treated in a primary care setting. Studies have shown that educational efforts and close cooperation between psychiatrists and general practitioners (GP's) lead to an increase in the proportion of depressed patients that are identified and properly treated. The use of diagnostic self-reports can facilitate this process for the GP. It is crucial to identify and treat the disorder early on, in order to improve prognosis, decrease the risk of complications and reduce costs for society and the health care system.

Although depression can be a feature of acute psychosis and an aftermath of a psychotic episode (post psychotic depression), data indicate that depressive syndromes in schizophrenia can be found years after the immediate post acute phase. Researchers acknowledge the clinical importance of recognizing that depressive symptoms are frequently described in patients diagnosed with schizophrenia. Using the framework of Antonovsky's (1972, 1987, 1992) Sense of Coherence as a guide, the article of Menzies (2000) explores what nurses can do to facilitate development of Generalized Resistance Resources (GRRs) in the physical, psychological, and emotional armamentarium of those diagnosed with schizophrenia, mood disorder not otherwise specified (NOS).

Alexander et al., (1999) administered a self-report measure of proneness to shame and guilt among 86 patients with moderate to severe depression, with the prediction that there would be a positive correlation of shame with severity of depression. But they found that guilt but not shame was associated with levels of depression. Shame-proneness demonstrated a unique association with a stable attributional style for negative outcomes, global negative self-evaluation, submissive behaviour and internalized anger.

King et al., (1997) studied the diagnostic Interview Schedule for Children (DISC-2.3) on a sample of 265 adolescent inpatients to determine type and concurrent validity of depressive symptoms and depressive disorder. The Children's Depression Rating Scale—Revised, Reynolds Adolescent Depression Scale (RADS), Suicide Ideation Questionnaire—Junior, Spectrum of Suicide Behaviour Scale, and clinical consensus diagnoses were used to assess concurrent validity. Results indicated that (1) parents, compared to adolescents, reported a higher prevalence of all depressive symptoms with the exception of weight change; (2) DISC-2.3 depressive and suicidal symptoms were related positively to independent validating criteria for all informant conditions, suggesting good concurrent validity; (3) the DISC-2.3 both informant condition correctly identified the most depressive disorders; and (4) the parent, but not the adolescent, DISC-2.3 Informant condition contributed to the prediction of clinical consensus diagnoses of depression after taking into account RADS scores.

In the year 1996, Power et al., conducted a study where they used Emotional Priming Paradigm [Power and Brewin (1990) Cogn. Emotion 4, 39-51] on a group of currently depressed patients and a group of non-depressed controls.

They revealed that the depressed patients showed significant facilitation effects on both the speed and rate of endorsement of negative trait adjectives when these were preceded by negative emotional primes. On the contrary the control subjects failed to show such facilitation effects.

Dysthymia (DD) may be thought of as depression associated with personality disorder, a phase in the pleomorphic natural history of unipolar depression or a result of exposure to chronic physical illness. Prevalence, clinical features, risk factors and prognosis may change with age. Beekman et al., (2004) conducted a study on large (n=3056) representative sample of elderly (55-85 years) in the Netherlands. They collected data on 277 depressed elderly to assess the 6 years prognosis of DD. The prevalence of DD (4.61%) was higher in women and it declined with age. The symptom profiles of DD and MDD were very similar. Those with DD were very likely to have had MDD earlier in life (44.0% in pure DD and 80.0% in those with double depression). The average age at onset (31 years) was earlier than in MDD (53 years). Environmental and personal vulnerability dominated the risk factors. Finally Beekman et al., (2004) concluded that although the prevalence declines with age, Dysthymia (DD) remains common in later life.

Gongora et al., (2004) attempted to carry out a research on personality disorders, depression, and coping styles in Argentinean bulimic patients. This study investigates the coping styles of bulimic patients with personality disorders (PDs) and the effects of the level of depression on the relations between PDs and coping covering 75 Argentinean bulimic outpatients engaged in treatment. They found no differences in the coping styles of bulimic patients with or without a personality disorder. When three specific PDs were considered—Avoidant, Obsessive-Compulsive, or Borderline PDs-clear differences in the coping styles of the bulimics were found. However, the differences disappeared when depression was controlled. Regarding the severity of the three specific PDs, coping styles were only found to be associated with the Avoidant PD. Depression showed to affect the relations between coping styles and two specific PDs-Avoidant and Borderline PDs-in bulimic patients.

Depressive episodes are significant in bipolar illness since patients can spend up to one-third of their lives in depression. Although the treatment of bipolar depression remains an understudied area, new data from randomized, controlled trials and naturalistic studies have expanded the range of treatments available. The main aim in the treatment of bipolar depression is the prevention of the patient switching to mania and cycle acceleration, and anti-depressant therapy may be contraindicated because of the risk for switching. Guidelines for the acute treatment of bipolar depression emphasize treatment with a mood stabilizer, of which lithium has been the most thoroughly studied in randomized, controlled trials in acute bipolar depression. Lamotrigine has also demonstrated significant efficacy in recent studies and has been approved by the FDA (Oral et al., 2004).

Dentists encounter numerous sources of professional stress, beginning in dental school. This stress can have a negative impact on their personal and professional lives. Dentists are prone to professional burnout, anxiety disorders and clinical depression, owing to the nature of clinical practice and the personality traits common among those who decide to pursue careers in dentistry. Many researchers suggest that to enjoy satisfying professional and personal lives, dentists must be aware of the importance of maintaining good physical and mental health (Rada RE, et al., 2004).

Depression typically begins in late adolescence or early adulthood, and the younger it starts the worse course there may be. US data on major depression by decade of age based on epidemiological study indicate that highest rate of current depression among the youngest group (6.1%), and the lowest rate among the oldest group (3.6%) (Burke, Burke, Regier, and Rae, 1990). Not only are the rates of onset and current depression highest among those in their late teens and early 20s, but several studies have now suggested an intriguing possibility: depression is on the increase among the young. Klerman and Weissman (1989) were among the first to note that rates of depressive disorder were relatively higher in those born more recently.

In addition to age differences in who is affected by depression, one of the most noteworthy characteristics of depression is that it is far more common among women than men (Weissman and Olfson, 1995). This apart, there are also indications that women's course of depression is different from men's. For example, women may have earlier onsets than men do (Sorenson et al., 1991).

Generally most depressive episodes clear up in 4-6 months even if not treated. However, most people who have had one episode will have another, and sometimes multiple recurrences, with about 25.0% developing chronic depression. Depression—even mild persistent depression—takes a severe toll on work, parental and marital relationships. The consequences of depression in terms of impaired functioning can set the stage for further depression in a self-perpetuating cycle.

So far as prevalence of different types of depression, there is no reliable published data. According to a review by Smith and Weissman (1992), the rates of current depression in various European countries ranged between 4.6-7.4%. In various US cities, rates based on the DSM criteria for major depression within the past six months were somewhat lower, ranging between 1.5-2.8%.

Most forms of psychological disorder affect individuals' interpersonal lives, impairing their social functioning by altering interpersonal behaviours and the quality of relating to others. Depression is no exception, because the symptoms of depression interfere with normal relationships. Sometimes depression is the cause of difficulties in interpersonal relationships. On the contrary, sometimes people suffer from depression as a result of interpersonal problems.

Difficulties in maintaining usual social transactions and discharging social responsibilities and relationships may be a key element of many depressions: disrupted social connectedness may cause depression, and depression disrupts relationships, potentially causing further depression. Negative early childhood experiences, in the form of insecure attachment relationships between parent and child and in learning maladaptive skills and cognitions, may contribute to vulnerability to depression. In fact, depression affects the family in adverse ways, especially contributing to marital discord, family burden, and poor adjustment in children.

Depressive people may have certain personality problems and behavioural traits that affect their relationships even when not depressed, including dependency, introversion and possibly, dysfunctional social skills and cognitions.

Findings of Jambunathan, Jaylakshmi (1992) indicate that lack of continued financial and emotional support from spouses and other family members can act as influencing factors in development of depression. Mitchell et al., 1993 found that only certain sub-dimensions of life satisfactions and withdrawal are related to depression.

Margo et al., (1993) in an attempt to compare defensive styles in depressed psychiatric patients could show that depressed men were more likely to use internalized defenses and the depressed women were more likely to use externalized defenses than their respective non-depressed comparison groups, showing thereby that there exists a relationship between depression severity and the amount of negatively biased self perception.

A number of studies have been carried out among children and adolescents in regard to their depression. While assessing depression among children, developmental considerations should be taken into account. For instance, irritability may be substituted for depressed mood because it is recognized both that irritability is a common expression of distress in depressed youngsters. According to recent study of dysthymic disorder in children, it differs from major depression primarily in the emphasis on gloomy thoughts and other negative affect, with fewer symptoms such as loss of interest, social withdrawal, fatigue, and reduced sleep and poor appetite (Kovacs, Akiskal, Gatsonis, and Parrone, 1994). Goodyer and Cooper (1993) found that 80.0% of their sample of 11-16 year-old girls with major depressive episode reported irritability, while Ryan et al., (1987) observed irritability or anger in 83.0% of a child and adolescent clinic sample.

Suicidal thoughts and attempts are among the diagnostic criteria for major depression. As many as half of the suicides in the United States are committed by people suffering from depression (Greenberg, 1982). Suicidal ideation is quite common in depressed youngsters, occurring in about two-thirds of pre-scholars, preadolescents, and adolescents (Mitchell et al., 1988; Ryan et al., 1987). Actual suicidal attempts occurred in 39.0% of the preadolescents and adolescent samples of Mitchell et al., (1988), with 6.0-12.0% of the Ryan et al., (1987) child and adolescent samples making moderate or severe attempts. These rates appear to be higher among depressed youngsters than among depressed adults.

Diagnosis of Depression

The present study covered depressive patients following DSM-IV criteria.

Justification of the Study

Literature indicates that not much study has been carried out among depressive patients to understand the personality dispositions, self-esteem, emotional control, and suicidal tendencies among depressive patients. This apart, the local Mental Health Care professionals working with depressive patients and the family members encounter different problems. For want of proper guidelines and sensitive screening tool for ascertaining suicidal tendencies among depressive patients sometimes they are unable to undertake a just-in-time early intervention programme for depressive patients in the family.

Hence the present study was aimed to carry out an investigation to understand the personality dimensions, self-esteem, emotional control, and suicidal tendencies among depressive patients. For ascertaining the suicidal tendencies and emotional control among depressive patients there was no locally adopted tests to meet the local needs. The present study adopted two new tests to understand suicidal tendencies and emotional control among depressive patients.

Objectives

To study the:

(1) Socio-economic and demographic background of depressive patients.
(2) Personality dispositions of depressive patients.
(3) Self-esteem of depressive patients.
(4) Emotional control of depressive patients.
(5) Suicidal tendencies of depressive patients.
(6) Perceived problems of family members in dealing with depressive patients, and
(7) To suggest need-based measures for family members for better care and management of depressive patients.

Hypotheses

(1) Personality dispositions of depressive patients and normal population of same age group differ significantly, irrespective of gender differences and chronicity of the disease.
(2) Personality dispositions of male and female depressive patients differ significantly, irrespective of age or chronicity of the disease.
(3) Personality dispositions of depressive patients differ significantly across chronicity of the disease, irrespective of gender.
(4) Self-esteem of depressive patients and normal population of same age group differs significantly, irrespective of gender differences and chronicity of the disease.
(5) Self-esteem of male and female depressive patients differs significantly, irrespective of age or chronicity of the disease.
(6) Self-esteem of depressive patients differs significantly across chronicity of the disease, irrespective of gender.
(7) Emotional control of depressive patients and normal population of same age group differs significantly, irrespective of gender differences and chronicity of the disease.

(8) Emotional control of male and female depressive patients differs significantly, irrespective of age or chronicity of the disease.

(9) Emotional control of depressive patients differs significantly across chronicity of the disease, irrespective of gender.

(10) Suicidal tendencies of depressive patients and normal population of same age group differ significantly, irrespective of gender differences and chronicity of the disease.

(11) Suicidal tendencies of male and female depressive patients differ significantly, irrespective of age or chronicity of the disease.

(12) Suicidal tendencies of depressive patients differ significantly across chronicity of the disease, irrespective of gender.

Operational Definition: In the present study patients of major depression and dysthymic depression were covered following DSM-IV criteria. However, in the following section, simple operational definition of all the key issues like depression, major depression, dysthymic depression, personality disposition, self-esteem, emotional control and Suicidal Tendencies have been provided below:

Depression: A mental state characterized by a pessimistic sense of inadequacy and a despondent lack of activity.

Major Depression: This is the most severe category of depression. In a major depression, more of the symptoms of depression are present, and they are usually more intense or severe. A major depression can result from a single traumatic event of our life, or may develop slowly as a consequence of numerous personal disappointments and life problems.

Dysthymic Depression: A type of depression involving long-term, chronic symptoms that are not disabling, but keep a person from functioning at 'full steam' or from feeling good. Dysthymia is a less severe type of depression than what is accorded the diagnosis of major depression. However, people with dysthymia may also sometimes experience major depressive episodes, suggesting that there is a continuum between dysthymia and major depression.

Personality Disposition: The term 'personality' refers to the total functions of an individual who interacts with his environment. In the present study the factors of 'personality disposition', which are explored, include introversion/ extroversion, self-concept, independence/dependence, temperament, adjustment and anxiety.

Self-esteem: Self-esteem can be defined as a positive feeling and respect for ourself. It is essentially a measure of self worth and importance. In the present study 'self-esteem' means socially perceived self of the individual i.e., individual's perception as to how the society perceives him/her.

Emotional Control: In the present study 'emotional control' means stress tolerance level of an individual.

Suicidal Tendencies: In the present study 'suicidal tendencies' means thoughts of self-destruction of an individual.

3

Methodology

Geographical Coverage

The present study was confined to Kolkata Metropolitan City and its suburbs.

Target Group

For the purpose of the present study the following categories of respondents were covered:

- Depressive patients, (Major Depressive and Dysthymic Depressive patients) irrespective of gender (selected following DSM-IV criteria).
- Normal population (matched group in terms of age, gender and education).
- Family members, either of the parents or guardian.

Study Tools

In order to achieve the objectives of the present study, following study tools were used:

Background Information Schedule developed by Dr. Sibnath Deb and Anjana Bhattacharjee (2002).

Multi-dimensional Personality Inventory developed by Km. Manju Agarwal (1988) and locally adapted by Anjana Bhattacharjee and Dr. Sibnath Deb (2002).

Self-esteem Inventory developed by M.S. Prasad and G.P.Thakur (1989) and locally adapted by Anjana Bhatacharjee and Dr.Sibnath Deb (2002).

Emotional Control Inventory developed by Samuel E. Krug (1989) and locally adapted by Anjana Bhattacharjee and Dr. Sibnath Deb (2002).

Suicidal Tendencies Inventory developed by Samuel E. Krug (1989) and locally adapted by Anjana Bhattacharjee and Dr. Sibnath Deb (2002).

Short Description of the Study Tools

Background Information Schedule

The Background Information Schedule was developed by Anjana Bhattacharjee and Dr. Sibnath Deb (2002) to gather information about socio-economic and familial background of the depressive patients. In addition, the schedule was also designed to gather information about the onset of the disease and the problems encountered by the family members in dealing with the patients and their suggestions thereof to deal with depressive patients more effectively. This schedule has three broad sections viz.,

Section 1: Socio-Economic and Treatment Related Information

This section has two parts. First part focuses on the demographic and socio-economic profile of the subject like age, sex, educational background, occupational status, monthly income, marital status, number of siblings and living environment (rural or urban area).

The second part designed to gather information about type of depression, onset of depressions, whether treatment received or not, any other physical complications and addiction related history of the depressive patients. Thus Section 1 consists of seventeen items.

Section 2: Family Related Information

This section consists of twelve items where main emphasis is given to gather information about the family background of the depressive patients for understanding both predisposing and precipitating factors of the disease. The main highlighting contents of this section are family history of depression, type of family, family environment, size of the family, interpersonal relationship among the family members, total family income, social network of the family, any major health problem in the family and addiction related history of the family members.

Section 3: Information Regarding Problems Perceived by the Family Members in Dealing with Depressive Patients

This section consists of nine items covering various problems encountered and perceived by the family members in dealing with the depressive patient. Also it reveals suicidal history of the patient and how the family members are deal with such crisis situations. This section also gathers information about social support available for the patient and what could be done for better management of the patient.

Multi-dimensional Personality Inventory

Description: The term 'Personality' refers to the total functions of an individual who interacts with his/her environment. The purpose of the measurement of personality is to describe a person in terms of traits. In the present study Multi-dimensional Personality Inventory was used to understand the personality dispositions of depressive patients.

The Multi-dimensional Personality Inventory was developed and standardized by Km Manju Agarwal in 1988. The inventory measures six dimensions of personality like extroversion-introversion, self-concept, dependence-independence, temperament, adjustment and anxiety. Each dimension has twenty items. Hence there are altogether 120 items in the inventory.

Response Mode: The response is recorded against three mode of response like 'yes', 'sometimes' and 'no'. The subject is instructed to put a tick (√) mark against the answer, which is best suited for him/her.

Scoring: The subject will get 3 score if answered 'yes', 2 score for answering 'sometimes' and 1 for answering 'no'.

Thus maximum score in each dimension is sixty and minimum score is twenty. There is no time limit for the completion of the inventory but generally the subject is asked to complete it as early as they can.

Reliability: For ascertaining the reliability coefficient of the inventory, it was administered to a sample of 600 students. The split-half reliability coefficient was computed for the six sub-scales as well as for the total score.

Table 3.1: Showing Split-Half Reliability Coefficient of the Inventory

Sub-Scale	*Correlation Coefficient*
• Extroversion-introversion	.82
• Self-concept	.84
• Dependence-independence.	.78
• Temperament.	.87
• Adjustment	.79
• Anxiety	.86
Total	.74

The Test-retest reliability of the inventory was also calculated following test-retest method on a sample of 100 students with an interval of 20 days. The test-retest reliability coefficient is given below:

Table 3.2: Showing Test-Retest Reliability Coefficient of the Inventory

Sub-Scale	*Correlation Coefficient*
• Extroversion-introversion	.72
• Self-concept	.81
• Dependence-independence	.69
• Temperament	.72
• Adjustment	.84
• Anxiety	.71
Total	.74

Validity: For ascertaining the validity, the scale was administered to a group of 100 students. The validity coefficient of the six sub-scales of this inventory is given in the next page:

Table 3.3: Showing Validity Coefficient of the Inventory

Sub-Scale	*Correlation Coefficient*
• Extroversion-introversion	.84
• Self-concept	.72
• Dependence-independence	.69
• Temperament	.84
• Adjustment	.82
• Anxiety	.76

Steps Followed for Local Adaptation of the Test

Step I: English version of the questionnaire was translated into easy Bengali language and again the same Bengali version of the questionnaire was retranslated into English to ensure proper translation of the same. It was checked by three subject experts. Translation from English to Bengali and retranslation to English version coincided i.e., the meaning of different items of the questionnaire of two versions remained same. This process was followed for ascertaining the face validity of the questionnaire.

Step II: For ascertaining the reliability, test-retest method was followed. The questionnaire was administered to the same group of population i.e., 100 normal population after 15 days of first administration and the reliability co-efficient was .79.

Self-esteem Inventory

Description: This inventory was developed and standardized by M.S. Prasad and G.P.Thakur (1989). According to them the self-evaluation of an individual not only depends upon how he perceives himself but also simultaneously depends upon the way he thinks about other's view regarding him. So they developed this inventory for measuring both the dimensions of self-esteem that is personally perceived and socially perceived self. Thus the inventory has two parts. Part one measures personally perceived self and part two measures socially perceived self. In the present study the second part of the inventory i.e., socially perceived self is used, which has thirty items. Of the thirty items, 17 are socially desirable and 13 are socially undesirable.

Response Mode: There are 7 possible response to each item/statement i.e. totally correct, correct to a large extent, partially correct, uncertain, partially wrong, wrong to a large extent and totally wrong. The respondents were asked to read each item carefully and to put a tick (√) mark against that response which is most appropriate for him.

Scoring: The items, which are socially desirable, would get 7 scores if answered completely 'true' and 1 if answered completely 'false'. Other intermediate answers would get scores accordingly. The socially undesirable items would score in the opposite manner i.e., the completely false point would get 7 scores and the completely true would get 1 score. Thus the maximum score of this inventory is 210 and minimum score is 30. Here low score indicates poor self-esteem while high score indicates high self-esteem.

Reliability: The two sets of inventory were administered to a sample of 400 students for ascertaining reliability coefficient. The split-half reliability coefficient of both the sets of inventory was found .82 and .78 for personally perceived self and socially perceived self respectively. Of the 400 students, 150 students were administered the two sets of inventory again after a gap of six weeks for evaluating test-retest reliability and reliability coefficients were found .69 and .66 respectively for personally perceived self and socially perceived self.

Validity: For ascertaining the validity, the scale was administered to a group of 200 students. The validity coefficient of the inventory was .84.

Steps Followed for Local Adaptation of the Test

Step I: English version of the questionnaire was translated into easy Bengali language and again the same Bengali version of the questionnaire was retranslated into English to ensure proper translation of the same. It was checked by three subject experts. Translation from English to Bengali and retranslation to English version coincided i.e., the meaning of different items of the questionnaire of two versions remained same. This process was followed for ascertaining the face validity of the questionnaire.

Step II: For ascertaining the reliability, test-retest method was followed. The questionnaire was administered to the same group of population i.e., 100 normal population after 15 days of first administration and the reliability co-efficient was .89.

Emotional Control Inventory

Description: This inventory is a part of Clinical Analysis Questionnaire (CAQ) developed by Samuel E Krug (1989).

Clinical Analysis Questionnaire was developed to meet the need of single instrument, as this could simultaneously measure both normal and pathological trait levels and provide full multi-dimensional profile of the individual. The test has 28 scales, 16 of which are the normal personality traits previously included in the 16 P.F, seven of which measures various primary manifestation of depression and five of which were developed to measure factors analytically identified traits that were discovered in the MMPI item pool. Consequently, the Clinical Analysis Questionnaire combines evidence of pathology along with information on personality structure itself. It thereby serves both diagnostic and treatment—planning function simultaneously.

The Clinical Analysis Questionnaire has 272 items, 128 in part 1 of the test, which covers the normal personality structure, and 144 in part II of the test, which covers the depression and pathological traits.

In the present study 2 sub-scales of Clinical Analysis Questionnaire i.e., emotional stability (FAC-C) and suicidal depression (FAC-D2) of depressive patient were used after local adaptation and ascertaining the reliability and validity of the scales.

The Emotional Control Inventory measures the normal personality trait i.e. Emotional Stability (FAC-C). This inventory finds the individuals stress tolerance level. There are altogether 15 items in the inventory. The higher the score on Factor C, the more resources the individual has available to meet the challenges of the day. FAC-C is also important in accident proneness, with low scoring individuals found to have significantly more accidents than high scoring individuals. This trait has been shown to have very consistent relationships with physical illness, especially coronary problems.

Clinically, low scores on this trait are especially important. The low scoring individual is typically overwhelmed by the challenges of the day. This inability to 'roll with the punches' (Skidmore, 1977) may be a precursor of other clinical evaluations in the CAQ profile. Cattell et al., (1970) and Karson and O'Dell (1976) have noted that the prognosis for therapeutic outcome is generally poorer when scores on this trait are low.

Response Mode: The responses are recorded against three point scale i.e., 'yes', 'sometimes' or 'uncertain' and 'no'. The subject is instructed to put a tick (√) mark against the answer, which is best suited for him/her.

Scoring: The maximum score of this inventory is 45 and minimum score is 15. High-scoring individuals are generally able to reach the personal goals without particular difficulty. They do not seem to be easily distracted when working on something. They frequently report general satisfaction with the way they have lived their lives. The high scoring individuals are emotionally stable and calm. Low score indicates less emotional control while high score indicates more emotional control.

The English version of this questionnaire was translated into easy Bengali language and three experts ascertained the face validity. Scoring was done according to the scoring manual.

Reliability and Validity: The reliability coefficient and validity coefficient of this scale were .83 and .75 respectively.

Steps Followed for Local Adaptation of the Test

Step I: English version of the questionnaire was translated into easy Bengali language and again the same Bengali version of the questionnaire was retranslated into English to ensure proper translation of the same. It was checked by three subject experts. Translation from English to Bengali and retranslation to English version coincided i.e., the meaning of different items of the questionnaire of two versions remained same. This process was followed for ascertaining the face validity of the questionnaire.

Step II: For ascertaining the reliability, test-retest method was followed. The questionnaire was administered to the same group of population i.e., 40 depressive patients after 15 days of first administration and the reliability co-efficient was .76.

Suicidal Tendencies Inventory

Description: This inventory is also a part of Clinical Analysis Questionnaire (CAQ) developed by Samuel E. Krug (1989). This inventory measures the pathological trait i.e. suicidal depression (FAC-D). In total there are 18 items in this inventory. The item contents of this inventory centres around thoughts of self-destruction.

Response Mode: There are three possible responses against each item/statement i.e., 'yes', 'sometimes'/'uncertain' and 'no'. The subject is instructed to put a tick (√) mark against the answer, which is best suited for him/her.

Scoring: The maximum score of this inventory is 45 and minimum score is 15. Low score indicates higher suicidal tendency while high score indicates lower suicidal tendency. The individual who scores low in this inventory indicates that he/she is disgusted with life, that life has become empty and meaningless for him/her. He/she entertains thought of death as a viable alternative of his/her present, hopeless situation.

The English version of this questionnaire was translated into easy Bengali language and three experts ascertained the face validity. Scoring was done following the scoring rational of the inventory.

Reliability and Validity: The reliability coefficient and Validity coefficient of this scale were .74 and .59 respectively.

Steps Followed for Local Adaptation of the Test

Step I: **English version of the questionnaire was translated into easy Bengali language and again the same Bengali version of**

the questionnaire was retranslated into English to ensure proper translation of the same. It was checked by three subject experts. Translation from English to Bengali and retranslation to English version coincided i.e., the meaning of different items of the questionnaire of two versions remained same. This process was followed for ascertaining the face validity of the questionnaire.

Step II: For ascertaining the reliability, test-retest method was followed. The questionnaire was administered to the same group of population i.e., 40 depressive patients after 15 days of first administration and the reliability co-efficient was .72.

Selection of Sample

The steps, which were followed for selection of sample, are as follows:

Step I: First, a list of Government Hospitals with Psychiatric Department and Private Health Centres with treatment facilities for mental patients were prepared in Kolkata. From the said two lists four centers, following two Government Hospitals and two Private Health Centres were selected randomly.

Government Hospitals

- R.G.Kar Medical College & Hospital.
- Calcutta Medical College & Hospital.

Private Mental Health Centres

- 'BaulMon'—A Centre for Human Mind, Jadavpur
- 'Antara'—A Centre for mental patients, Baruipur

Step II: From the said four Mental Health Centres, altogether 118 depressive patients (48 were suffering from Major Depression while the rest 70 were suffering from Dysthymic Depression) were covered in the study. Among them 63 were male and 55 were female. They were selected from the Government Hospitals and two Private Mental Health Centres following incidental sampling technique.

Step III: A group of 118 normal population comprised of 63 male and 55 female population were covered in this study and they were selected purposively when they came with the patients for treatment in the said four mental health centres, two Government Hospitals and two Private Mental Health Centres. Normal sample were matched in terms of gender, age, and education.

Step IV: In addition, a group of 118 family members-53 life partners, 45 fathers and 20 mothers were covered in the study to have their views about the problems encountered by them in dealing with the depressive patients and they were selected purposively. In short, the sample structure is given below:

Table 3.4: Sample Structure

Respondents	*Number*
• Depressive patients	118
• Normal population (matched group)	118
• Family Members	118
Total	354

Data Collection

First, permission from the authorities of two Hospitals and two private Mental Health Centres was obtained and then a tentative time schedule was developed in consultation with the authorities of the said health centres for data collection.

Data were collected from the depressive patients following face-to-face interview method while in case of semi-literate and illiterate normal population the same method was followed. But in case of normal educated population self-administration method was employed.

First, rapport was established with the patients after having casual discussion about their likings, disliking and hobbies and then the objectives of the study was explained and how the findings could be beneficial for the people like them so that they feel comfortable and relaxed while sharing necessary personal information and/or responding to different items of the psychological tests.

Depressive patients were selected following DSM IV criteria. In case of any confusion concerned psychiatrists were consulted. Altogether 130 depressive patients were contacted. But finally 118 participated in the study voluntarily. For collection of data from normal population, they were briefed about the objectives of the study and data were collected from those who voluntarily agreed to participate in the study. Normal population was contacted in the Hospital premises and/or in the private clinics. For collection of data from the family members especially from father, mother or guardian they were approached, while they came to Health Centres/ Private Clinics with the depressive patient.

Data Analysis

Data collected from the depressive patients and normal population were checked and edited so that any gap or confusion identified at the preliminary stage could be clarified henceforth. The filled in data sheets were subjected to in-house through editing and scrutiny. Finally, the data from the data sheets were entered with accuracy and precision into the computer for computational purpose.

Statistics is the science of methodology for the collection, systematic presentation, mathematical analysis and interpretation of data and for drawing inferences about the explored property in the relevant population.

For statistical analysis of the data the SYSTAT statistical package was used. In case of quantitative data descriptive statistics like measures of Central Tendency and dispersions were carried out and then 't'-test was applied for verification of the research hypotheses.

For analysis of qualitative data content analysis was carried out.

Ethical Issues Considered

Success of any study depends upon wholehearted cooperation from the respondents. If the respondents are not willing to participate in the study voluntarily they might provide haphazard response, which could mislead the overall findings of the study. In order to ensure the quality data and also for ethical purposes the following steps were adopted:

- Objectives of the study were briefed to all the study subjects.
- Informed consent was obtained.
- Confidentiality of information was ensured.
- Subject was asked that they could withdraw themselves during the study period if they wish.

Problems Encountered

While doing any studies every researcher face some problems and accordingly they find out the solutions to achieve their objectives. It is important to describe the problems encountered by any investigator so that future researchers can learn from the same and adopt proper measures accordingly for doing the similar study in future more effectively.

In this study also the researcher faced a number of problems. The main problem encountered by the investigator included sustaining the interest of some of the depressive patients for data collection.

Some of the respondents, both normal and depressive patients became restless after giving data for one/two tests. In that case researcher fixed up another date as per convenience of the respondents. In some cases researcher visited the house of the respondents if it was located within a reasonable distance.

Convincing some of the family members to share the problems encountered by them in dealing with the depressive patient was really a difficult task. Some of the family members did not agree to spare sometime from their busy schedule.

Hence researcher had to fix up another appointment for data collection from the family members.

Sometimes it was difficult to convince the general population for voluntary participation in this research work.

Non-availability of respondents despite the appointment. Some of the respondents especially the patient parties did not turn up on the date of appointment.

Sometime researcher had to wait for a long time to meet the patient in the Government Hospitals because of patient load.

Sometimes it was very difficult to make understand the meaning of the statements to some illiterate subjects (both depressive patients and normal subjects).

Limitations of the Study

In some study it is very difficult to get adequate number of sample and/or to obtain the consent for voluntarily participation in the study. In this study also researcher faced the same problem. The study was carried out covering only 118 depressive patients. To reconfirm the verified hypotheses another study with larger sample is suggested.

4

Interpretation of Results

In order to achieve the objectives of the present study, data were collected from 118 depressive patients, 118 normal population and 118 family members. After thorough scrutiny and editing of the data necessary statistical treatment was done for verification of the hypotheses. Data were presented under three broad sections as follows:

- *Section I*: Demographic and Socio-economic Information,
- *Section II*: Mental Dispositions of the Depressive Patients,
- *Section III*: Health Seeking Behaviour, Perceived Problems and Solutions.

Section I: Demographic and Socio-economic Information

Data pertaining to demographic and socio-economic information about the depressive patients have been provided in Table 4.1 Depressive patients came from all age groups. Findings of the present study indicate that depression mostly affected people over 20 years of age.

Out of a total of 118 depressive patients 63 (53.4%) were male while the rest 55 (46.6%) were female (Fig.4.1).

So far as educational background is concerned, most of the depressive patients were found to be Under Graduates while 14.4% and 16.9% depressive patients were Graduates and Post Graduates respectively (Fig.4.2).

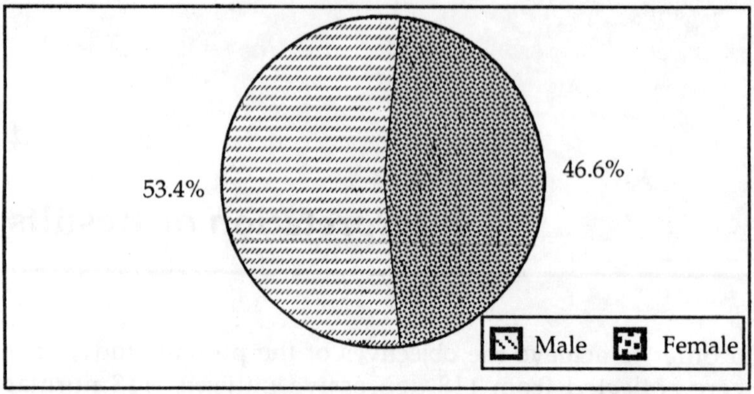

Fig. 4.1: Gender Distribution of the Depressive Patients

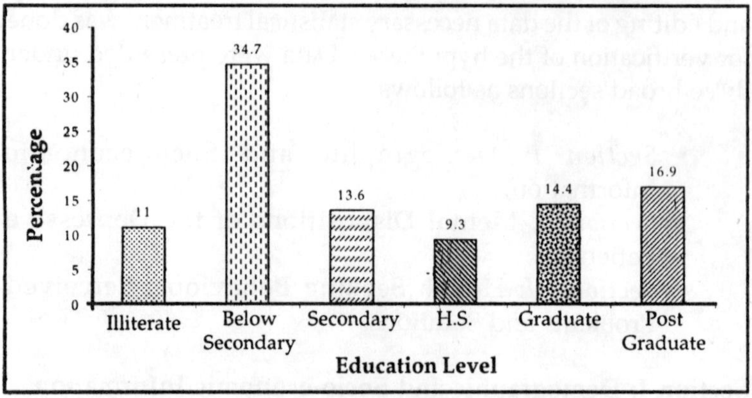

Fig. 4.2: Level of Education of the Depressive Patients

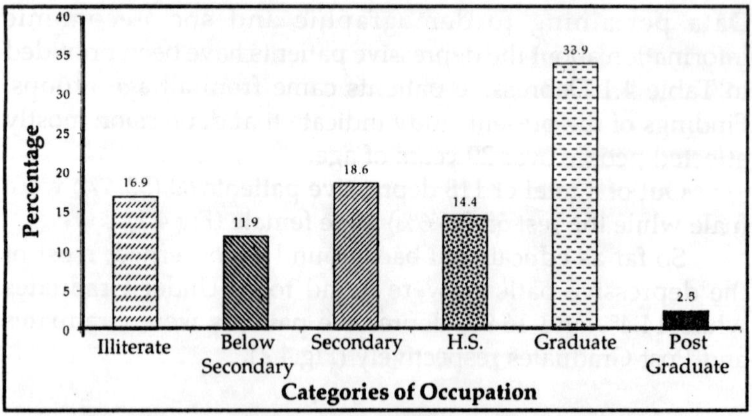

Fig. 4.3: Occupational Pattern of the Depressive Patients

Male depressive patients were mostly found to be in service (16.9%) and business (11.9%), while female depressive patients were housewife (33.9%). In addition, 18.6% were unemployed while 14.4% were students (Fig.4.3).

So far as marital status is concerned, 38.1% were married while the rest 23.7, 16.9 and 21.2% were single, divorcee/ separated and widowed respectively (Fig.4.4).

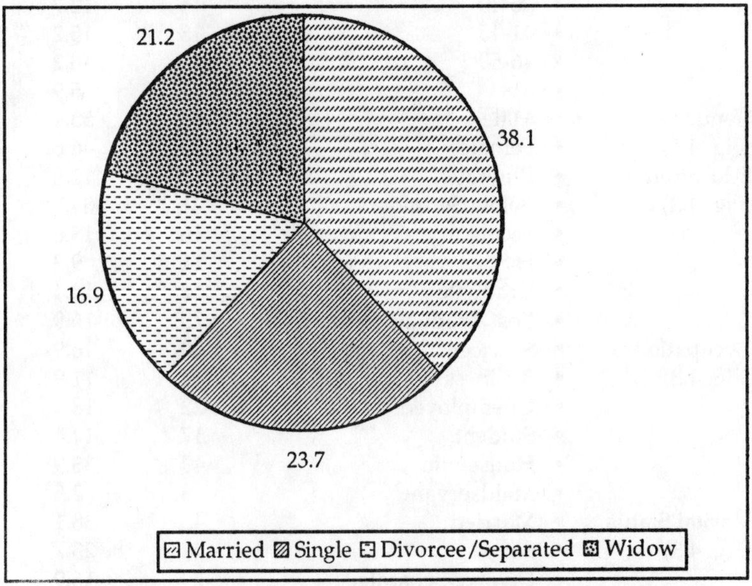

Fig. 4.4: Marital Status of the Depressive Patients

Majority of the depressive patients (59.3%) were found to have no source of income especially the female depressive patients while the rest 10.2, 8.5, 5.9, 12.7 and 3.4% earn below Rs.4000, Rs. 4001-8000, Rs.8001-12000, Rs.12001-16000 and above Rs.16001 per month respectively (Table 4.1).

Table 4.1: Demographic and Socio-economic Information

Parameters	*Characteristics*	*Mode of Response*	
		Frequency	*Percentage*
Age	• Below 20	4	3.4
	• 21-25	20	16.9
	• 26-30	24	20.3
	• 31-35	18	15.3
	• 36-40	15	12.7
	• 41-45	18	15.2
	• 46-50	12	10.2
	• 51+	7	5.9
Gender	• Male	63	53.4
(Fig. 4.1)	• Female	55	46.6
Education	• Illiterate	13	11.0
(Fig. 4.2)	• Below Secondary	41	34.7
	• Secondary	16	13.6
	• H.S.	11	9.3
	• Graduate	17	14.4
	• Post Graduate	20	16.9
Occupation	• Service	20	16.9
(Fig. 4.3)	• Business	14	11.9
	• Unemployed	22	18.6
	• Student	17	14.4
	• Housewife	40	33.9
	• Maidservant	3	2.5
Marital Status	• Married	45	38.1
(Fig. 4.3)	• Single	28	23.7
	• Divorce/Separated	20	16.9
	• Widow	25	21.2
Income of the	• No Income	70	59.3
Subject	• Below Rs. 4000	12	10.2
	• Rs. 4001-8000	10	8.5
	• Rs. 8001-12000	7	5.9
	• Rs. 12001-16000	15	12.7
	• Rs. 16001 and above	4	3.4

Base: All Respondents.

About two-fifth (40.7%) of the patients were suffering from depression for the last one year while the rest were suffering from the same mental health problem for more than last one year (Table 4.3).

Table 4.2: Duration, Types of Depression and Treatment

Parameters	*Characteristics*	*Mode of Response*	
		Frequency	*Percentage*
Duration (N=118)	• For the last I year	48	40.7
	• For more than 1 year	70	59.3
Types of Depression (N=118) Fig.4.5	• Major Depression	48	40.7
	• Dysthymic Depression	70	59.3
Whether Received any Treatment (N=118)	• Yes	95	80.5
	• No	23	19.5
If yes, whether benefited (N=95)	• Fully benefitted	25	26.3
	• Partially benefitted	33	34.7
	• Not at all benefitted	29	30.5
	• Difficult to comment	8	8.4

Out of a total of 118 depressive patients covered in the study, 40.7% were found to be patients of Major Depression while 59.3% were suffering from Dysthymic Depression (Table 4.2). Already 80.5% depressive patients had received some sort of treatment while 19.5% yet to receive any such treatment (Fig.4.5).

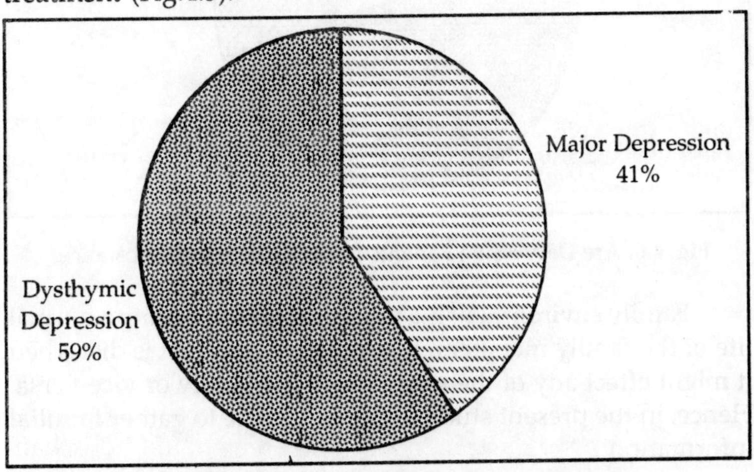

Fig. 4.5: Types of Depression among the Patients

Out of 95 depressive patients who received treatment, family members of 25 (26.3%) depressive patients stated that they have been fully benefited, 33 (34.7%) family members benefited partially while 29 (30.5%) stated that they are not at all benefited (Table 4.2).

Replying to a question whether the subject suffered or have been suffering from any major health problem, 27 (22.7%) stated 'yes'. The health problem from which they suffered and/or were suffering included cancer (8/27), diabetics (2/27), cardiovascular disorder (11/27) and others like liver problem, asthma etc. Most of the depressive patients were suffering from the same health problem for more than last one year (Table 4.3). Out of 118 depressive patients, 35 (29.7%) depressive patients were found to be dependent on mind-altering substances. The types of health problems and addition problems have been provided in Table 4.3 (Fig. 4.6).

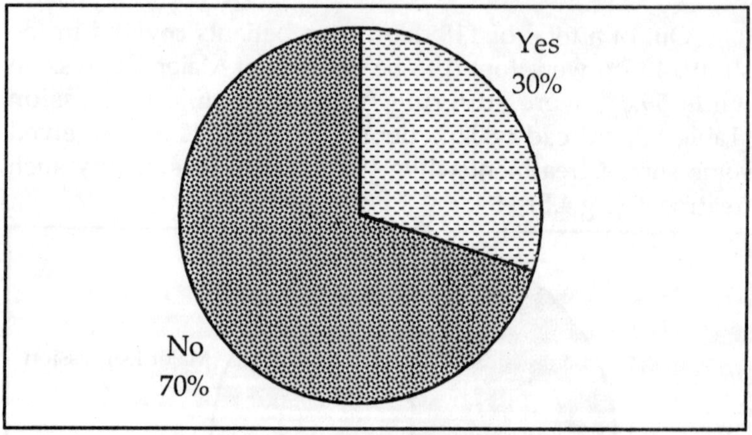

Fig. 4.6: Are Depressive Patients Dependent on any Substance?

Family environment is a crucial factor for leading a normal life of the family members. If family environment is disturbed it might effect any of the members of the family or vice versa. Hence, in the present study effort was made to gather familial information.

Table 4.3: Information Pertaining to Health Problem and Addition Problem of the Depressive Patients

Parameters	*Characteristics*	*Mode of Response*	
		Frequency	*Percentage*
Whether subject suffered from any major health problem (N=118)	• Yes	27	22.9
	• No	91	77.1
If yes, what health problems (N=27)	• Cancer	8	29.6
	• Diabetics	2	7.4
	• Cardiovascular	11	40.7
	• Others	6	22.2
For how long (N=27)	• For the last I year	6	22.2
	• For more than 1 year	21	77.8
Whether subject dependent on any substance (N=118)	• Yes	35	29.7
	• No	83	70.3
If yes, dependent on what substance (N=35)	• Alcohol	16	45.7
	• Sleeping Tablets	3	8.6
	• Narcotic Drugs	7	20.0
	• Others	9	25.7

Data pertaining to familial information have been depicted in Table 4.4. It has been observed that about one-fifth (21.2%) of the depressive patients have family history of depression and an overwhelming number of depressive patients came from single family (87.3%) with small family size i.e., more than 50.0% of the depressive patients came from family with less than 4 members (Table 4.4).

So far as family environment is concerned, it has been observed that the family environment of 42.3 and 28.0% depressive patients were 'not so peaceful' and 'disturbed' (Fig. 4.7).

The total monthly income of the depressive patients indicates that most of them belonged to middle class families (Table 4.4). In case of more than one-third (38.1%) of the depressive patients the social network was found to be low (Fig. 4.8).

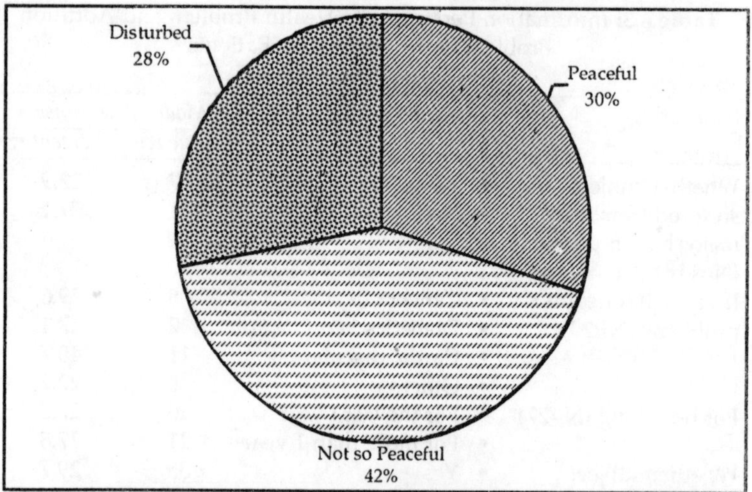

Fig. 4.7: Family Environment of the Depressive Patients

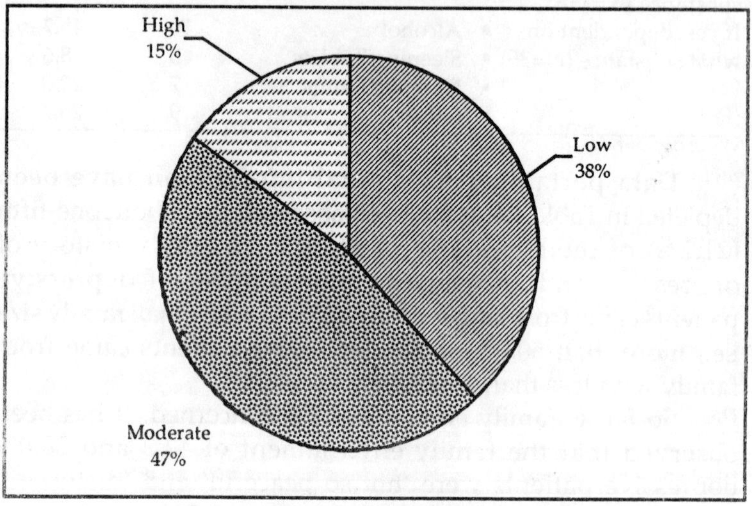

Fig. 4.8: Social Network of the Family

In case of 25 depressive patients (21.2%) there was a history of physical illness in the family and in case of most of the families they were suffering from some major health problems for more than one year.

Table 4.4: Family Related Information

Parameters	*Characteristics*	*Mode of Response*	
		Frequency	*Percentage*
Any Family History of Depression (N=118)	• Yes	25	21.2
	• No	93	78.8
Type of Family (N=118)	• Joint	15	12.7
	• Single	103	87.3
Family Size (N=118)	• < 4 members	70	59.3
	• 4-6 members	33	28.0
	• 7 and above	15	12.7
Family Environment (N=118) Fig. 4.7	• Peaceful	35	29.7
	• Not so peaceful	50	42.3
	• Disturbed	33	28.0
Total Income of the Family in a Month (N=118)	• Below Rs.4000	12	11.2
	• 4001-8000	35	29.7
	• 8001-12000	38	32.2
	• 12001-16000	15	12.7
	• 16001 and above	18	15.3
Social Network of the Family (N=118) (Fig. 4.8)	• Low social network	45	38.1
	• Moderate social network	55	46.6
	• High social network	18	15.3
Whether any family member suffering from any health problem?	• Yes	25	21.2
	• No	93	78.8
If yes, for how long (N=25)	• For the last 1 year	4	15.0
	• For more than 1 year	21	84.0

Section II: Mental Dispositions of the Depressive Patients

Personality Dispositions

For understanding the personality dispositions of the depressive patients and for comparison of the same with the normal population, Multi-dimensional Personality Inventory was used after local adaptation, which is a standardized psychological test. The distribution of measures of central tendency and deviations have been provided in Table 4.5.

Table 4.5: Central Tendency Measures and Deviations of Data Collected Through Personality Dispositions Inventory

Sub-scales	*Sample Group*	*Central Tendency Measures*			*Deviations*	
		Mean	*Median*	*Mode*	*SD*	*SK*
Introversion/ Extroversion	• Depressive Patients	30.57	29	25.56	7.65	1.10
	• Normal Population	42.44	45	50.12	9.77	-0.57
Self-concept	• Depressive Patients	30.94	31	31.12	5.58	0.15
	• Normal Population	38.33	39	40.34	6.65	-0.57
Dependence/ Independence	• Depressive Patients	33.09	33	32.82	5.75	0.15
	• Normal Population	42.10	44	47.8	6.38	-0.55
Temperament	• Depressive Patients	37.49	37	36.02	6.60	0.06
	• Normal Population	40.18	40	39.64	7.22	0.03
Adjustment	• Depressive Patients	35.85	35	33.3	5.91	0.35
	• Normal Population	42.32	46	53.36	6.88	-0.61
Anxiety	• Depressive Patients	45.08	46	47.84	5.44	-0.46
	• Normal Population	39.49	38	35.02	7.75	0.33

The mean value of the depressive patients with regard to personality variables like extroversion/introversion, self-concept, independence/dependence, temperament and adjustment was found to be 30.57, 30.94, 33.09, 37.49 and 35.85 respectively which were lesser than the mean value of normal population with respect to the same personality variables i.e., 42.44, 38.33, 42.10, 40.18 and 42.32 respectively. However, with regard to anxiety it has been observed that the mean value of depressive patients was more (45.08) than that of their counterparts (39.49), which indicates that the depressive patients suffer from more anxiety. The standard deviations of scores of the said personality variables of the depressive patients was 7.65, 5.58, 5.75, 6.60, 5.91 and 5.44 while in case of normal population it was 9.77, 6.65, 6.38, 7.22, 6.88 and 7.75 respectively.

The data were then processed properly for the verification of the first hypothesis i.e.,

> *'Personality dispositions of depressive patients and normal population of same age group differ significantly, irrespective of gender differences and chronicity of the disease.'*

To verify the above hypothesis 't'-test was applied for comparing the means and standard deviations as displayed in Table 4.5.

From Table 4.6, it has been observed that 't'-values are significant (p<. 01) in case of all the personality variables viz., extroversion/introversion, self-concept, independence/dependence, temperament, adjustment and anxiety.

Hence, it may be stated that first hypothesis i.e., 'personality dispositions of depressive patients and normal population of same age group differ significantly, irrespective of gender differences and chronicity of the disease', is retained.

Therefore, it may be stated that depressive patients are more introvert, possess low self-concept, more dependent on others, short tempered, low adjustment capacity and more anxious than their normal counterparts with respect to the said personality variables (Table 4.6).

The data were then processed again for the verification of the second hypothesis i.e.,

> *'Personality dispositions of male and female depressive patients differ significantly, irrespective of age or chronicity of the disease'.*

In order to confirm the above hypothesis 't'-test was applied for comparing the means and standard deviations as displayed in Table 4.7.

From Table 4.7, it has been observed that 't'-values of male and female depressive patients were found to be insignificant in case of four personality variables viz., extroversion/ introversion ($p > .05$), self-concept ($p > .05$), independence/ dependence ($p > .05$), and anxiety ($p > .05$). However in case of temperament 't' value was significant at .05 level ($p < .05$) and in case of adjustment variable 't' value was significant at .01 level ($p < .01$).

Table 4.6: Comparison of Sub-Scales of Personality Dispositions of Depressive Patients and Normal Population

Sub-scales	*Sample Group*	*Number*	*Mean*	*S.D.*	*'t' Value*	*Level of Significance*
Introversion/ Extroversion	• Depressive Patients	118	29	7.65	10.89	$p < .01$
	• Normal Population	118	45	9.77		
Self-concept	• Depressive Patients	118	31	5.58	9.93	$p < .01$
	• Normal Population	118	39	6.65		
Dependence/ Independence	• Depressive Patients	118	33	5.75	11.83	$p < .01$
	• Normal Population	118	44	6.38		
Temperament	• Depressive Patients	118	37	6.60	2.82	$p < .01$
	• Normal Population	118	40	7.22		
Adjustment	• Depressive Patients	118	35	5.91	13.54	$p < .01$
	• Normal Population	118	46	6.88		
Anxiety Extroversion	• Depressive Patients	118	46	5.44	-8.03	$p < .01$
	• Normal Population	118	38	7.75		

Hence, it may be stated that second hypothesis i.e., personality dispositions of male and female depressive patients differ significantly, irrespective of age or chronicity of the disease has been accepted only in case of two personality variables as mentioned above.

However, it has been observed that the mean scores for the male depressive patients were greater in case of all the personality variables as compared to female depressive patients.

So, from the mean scores it can be stated that male depressive patients possessed high self-concept, they were more adjusted, more independent as well as more anxious than their counterparts while female depressive patients were more introvert and short tempered as compared to their male counterparts.

Table 4.7: Comparison of Sub-scales of Personality Dispositions of Male and Female Depressive Patients

Sub-scales	*Depressive Patients*	*Number*	*Mean*	*S.D.*	*'t' Value*	*Level of Significance*
Introversion/	• Male	63	31.36	7.95	0.725	$p > .05$
Extroversion	• Female	55	29.67	7.25		
Self-concept	• Male	63	31.43	5.26	0.676	$p > .05$
	• Female	55	30.40	5.90		
Dependence/	• Male	63	34.15	5.30	1.671	$p > .05$
Independence	• Female	55	31.87	5.80		
Temperament	• Male	63	38.68	7.43	2.299	$p > .05$
	• Female	55	36.12	5.23		
Adjustment	• Male	63	37.46	6.18	2.670	$p > .01$
	• Female	55	34.01	5.03		
Anxiety	• Male	63	45.14	5.49	-0.70	$p > .05$
	• Female	55	45.01	5.43		

For verification of third hypothesis as stated below data were processed accordingly and is provided in Table 4.8.

'Personality dispositions of depressive patients differ significantly across chronicity of the disease, irrespective of gender'.

To check the above hypothesis, 't'-test was applied for comparing the means and standard deviations as displayed in Table 4.8.

From Table 4.8, it has been observed that 't'-values of two categories of depressive patients i.e., the patients who have been suffering from depression for the last one year and more than last one year were found to be significant in case of all the personality variables viz., extroversion/introversion, self-concept, independence/dependence, temperament, adjustment and anxiety.

Table 4.8: Comparison of Sub-scales of Personality Dispositions of Depressive Patients Suffering from this Mental Health Problem for the last one Year and more than one Year

Sub-scales	*Depressive Patients suffering from this Mental Health for the Last*	*Central Tendency Measures and Deviation*			*'t' Value*	*Level of Significance*
		Number	*Mean*	*S.D.*		
Introversion/ Extroversion	• One year	48	36.18	7.92	6.16	$p < .01$
	• More than one year	70	26.72	4.92		
Self-concept	• One year	48	35.43	3.96	7.28	$p < .01$
	• More than one year	70	28.01	4.43		
Dependence/ Independence	• One year	48	37.31	5.13	7.10	$p < .01$
	• More than one year	70	30.20	4.15		
Temperament	• One year	48	32.20	4.95	-8.79	$p < .01$
	• More than one year	70	42.11	4.94		
Adjustment	• One year	48	39.14	5.44	4.88	$p < .01$
	• More than one year	70	33.60	5.13		
Anxiety	• One year	48	37.31	5.13	-2.715	$p < .01$
	• More than one year	70	30.20	4.15		

Hence, it may be stated that the third hypothesis i.e., 'personality dispositions of depressive patients differ significantly across chronicity of the disease, irrespective of gender' has been accepted.

However, the mean score was greater with regard to introversion/extroversion, self-concept, dependence/independence, adjustment and anxiety in case of depressive patients who were suffering from depression for the last one year as compared to depressive patients who were suffering from depression for more than one year. It means that the depressive patients who were suffering from depression for the last one year were less introvert, possessed high self-concept, more independent, well adjusted as well as more anxious in comparison to those who were suffering from depression for more than one year. On the other hand, the second category of depressive patients was more introvert and good tempered than those of their counterparts.

Self-esteem

In order to understand the self-esteem of the depressive patients and for comparison of the same with the normal population, 'Self-esteem Inventory'—a standardized psychological test was used after local adaptation. After ascertaining the face validity and socio-cultural admissibility of the same reliability of the test was also ascertained. The distribution of measures of central tendency and deviations have been provided in Table 4.9.

Table 4.9: Central Tendency Measures and Deviations of Data Collected Through Self-esteem Inventory

Sample Group	*Central Tendency Measures*			*Deviations*	
	Mean	*Median*	*Mode*	*SD*	*SK*
Depressive Patients	30.94	31	31.12	5.51	0.15
Normal Population	38.33	39	40.34	6.65	-0.74

The mean value of the depressive patients with regard to self-esteem was 30.94, which was lesser than the mean value of normal population (38.33). It indicates that depressive patients possessed lower self-esteem as compared to normal population. The standard deviation of the scores of self-esteem of depressive patients was 5.51 while it was 6.65 in case of normal population.

The data were then processed properly for the verification of the fourth hypothesis i.e.,

'Self-esteem of depressive patients and normal population of same age group differs significantly, irrespective of gender differences and chronicity of the disease'.

In order to validate the above hypothesis 't'-test was applied for comparing the means and standard deviations of depressive patients and normal population with regard to self-esteem variable as displayed in Table 4.10.

It has been observed that 't'-value was significant (p <. 01) in case of self-esteem. Therefore, it may be stated that the fourth hypothesis i.e., 'self-esteem of depressive patients and normal population of same age group differ significantly, irrespective of gender differences and chronicity of the disease' is retained.

Table 4.10: Comparison of Self-esteem of Depressive Patients and Normal Population

Sample Group	*Number*	*Mean*	*S.D.*	*'t' Value*	*Level of Signi-ficance*
Depressive Patients	118	30.94	5.51	10.29	p < .01
Normal Population	118	38.33	6.65		

For verification of fifth hypothesis as given below, the data were processed accordingly and is presented in Table 4.11.

'Self-esteem of male and female depressive patients differs significantly, irrespective of age or chronicity of the disease'.

The verification of the above hypothesis was made possible by application of't'-test.

It has been observed that 't'-value was significant ($p < .01$) in case of self-esteem variable. Hence, it may be stated that the fifth hypothesis i.e., 'self-esteem of male and female depressive patients differs significantly, irrespective of age or chronicity of the disease' has been retained.

Table 4.11: Comparison of Self-esteem of Male and Female Depressive Patients

Sample Group	*Number*	*Mean*	*S.D.*	*'t' Value*	*Level of Significance*
Male Depressive Patients	63	31.42	5.26	3.48	p < .01
Female Depressive Patients	55	30.40	5.92		

The data were then processed for the verification of sixth hypothesis i.e.,

'Self-esteem of depressive patients differs significantly across chronicity of the disease, irrespective of gender'.

To ascertain the above hypothesis, 't'-test was applied for comparing the means and standard deviations of the depressive patients who were suffering from depression for the last one year and more than one year as displayed in Table 4.12.

It has been observed that the patients who were suffering from depression for the last one year and more than one year differed significantly ($p<.01$) in respect to self-esteem variable (Table 4.12). Hence, it may be stated that the sixth hypothesis i.e., 'self-esteem of depressive patients differs significantly across chronicity of the disease, irrespective of gender' is retained. From the mean score of the self-esteem it may be stated that the depressive patients who were suffering from depression for the last one year possessed high self-esteem as compared to their counterparts i.e., the depressive patients who were suffering from depression for more than last one year.

Table 4.12: Comparison of Self-esteem of Depressive Patients suffering from this Mental Health Problem for the Last One Year and More Than One Year

Depressive Patients (Suffering From this Mental Health for the Last)	*Number*	*Mean*	*S.D.*	*'t' Value*	*Level of Significance*
One year	48	35.43	3.96	5.51	$p < .01$
More than one year	70	28.01	4.43		

Emotional Control

Data pertaining to 'emotional control' of the depressive patients and for comparison of the same with the normal population was collected by 'Emotional Control Inventory'—a standardized psychological test which was further locally adapted. After ascertaining the face validity and socio-cultural admissibility of the same reliability of the test was also ascertained. The distribution of measures of central tendency and deviations have been provided in Table 4.13.

Table 4.13: Central Tendency Measures and Deviations of Data Collected Through Emotional Control Inventory

Sample Group	*Central Tendency Measures*			*Deviations*	
	Mean	*Median*	*Mode*	*SD*	*SK*
Depressive Patients	27.98	27	25.04	4.24	0.23
Normal Population	32.46	33	34.08	4.71	-0.44

The mean value of the depressive patients with regard to 'emotional control' was 27.98, which was lesser than the mean value of normal population i.e., 32.46. It indicates that depressive patients have less emotional control as compared to their normal counterparts. The standard deviation of the scores of 'emotional control' of depressive patients was 4.24 while in case of normal population it was 4.71.

The data were then processed for the verification of the seventh hypothesis i.e.,

'Emotional control of depressive patients and normal population of same age group differs significantly, irrespective of gender differences and chronicity of the disease'.

For verification of the above hypothesis 't'-test was applied with a view to comparing the means and standard deviations of depressive patients and normal population with regard to 'emotional control' variable as displayed in Table 4.14.

It has been observed that 't'-value was significant (p<. 01) in case of 'emotional control' variable. Therefore, it may be stated that the seventh hypothesis i.e., 'emotional control of depressive patients and normal population of same age group differ significantly, irrespective of gender differences and chronicity of the disease' has been accepted.

Table 4.14: Comparison of Emotional Control of Depressive Patients and Normal Population

Sample Group	*Number*	*Mean*	*S.D.*	*'t' Value*	*Level of Significance*
Depressive Patients	118	27.98	4.24	8.02	p < .01
Normal Population	118	32.46	4.71		

For verification of eighth hypothesis as given below, the data were processed accordingly and is presented in Table 4.15.

'Emotional control of male and female depressive patients differs significantly, irrespective of age or chronicity of the disease'.

To check the above hypothesis 't'-test was applied for comparing the means and standard deviations of the male and female depressive patients with regard to 'emotional control' variable as displayed in Table 4.15.

Table 4.15 reveals that male and female depressive patients differed significantly with respect to variable called 'emotional control' (p< .05). Hence, hypothesis eight i.e., 'emotional control of male and female depressive patients differs significantly, irrespective of age or chronicity of the disease' has been accepted.

Since the mean score of female depressive patients was lower as compared to male depressive patients it may be inferred that female depressive patients have less emotional control than those of male depressive patients (Table 4.15).

Table 4.15: Comparison of Emotional Control of Male and Female Depressive Patients

Sample Group	*Number*	*Mean*	*S.D.*	*'t' Value*	*Level of Signi-ficance*
Male Depressive Patients	63	28.90	3.91	2.45	p< .05
Female Depressive Patients	55	26.92	4.38		

For verification of ninth hypothesis as given below, the data were processed accordingly and presented in Table 4.16.

'Emotional control of depressive patients differs significantly across chronicity of the disease, irrespective of gender '.

To check the above hypothesis 't'-test was applied for comparing the means and standard deviations of the depressive patients who were suffering from depression for the last one year and more than one year as displayed in Table 4.16.

Table 4.16: Comparison of Emotional Control of Depressive Patients suffering from this Mental Health Problem for The Last One Year and More Than One Year

Depressive Patients Suffering From This Mental Health for the Last	*Number*	*Mean*	*S.D.*	*'t' Value*	*Level of Signi-ficance*
One Year	48	30.08	3.75	3.37	p< .01
More than One Year	70	26.68	4.16		

It has been observed that 't'-value was significant (p<. 01) in case of 'emotional control' variable. Hence, it may be stated that the ninth hypothesis i.e., emotional control of depressive patients differs significantly across chronicity of the disease, irrespective of gender differences' has been accepted. From the mean scores also, it is evident that the depressive patients who were suffering from depression for the last one year were emotionally more stable as compared to their counterparts.

Suicidal Tendencies

In order to understand the 'suicidal tendencies' among the depressive patients and for comparison of the same with the normal population 'Suicidal Tendencies Inventory' was used after local adaptation. The distribution of measures of central tendency and deviations have been provided in Table 4.17.

Table 4.17: Central Tendency Measures and Deviations of Data Collected Through Suicidal Tendencies Inventory

Sample Group	*Central Tendency Measures*			*Deviations*	
	Mean	*Median*	*Mode*	*SD*	*SK*
Depressive Patients	33.89	34	34.22	6.88	0.02
Normal Population	39.57	39.5	39.36	6.16	-0.17

The mean value of the depressive patients with regard to 'suicidal tendencies' was 33.89, which was lesser than the mean value of normal population i.e., 39.57. The standard deviation of the scores of 'suicidal tendencies' of depressive patients was 6.88 while in case of normal population it was 6.16.

The data were then processed for the verification of the tenth hypothesis i.e.,

'Suicidal tendencies of depressive patients and normal population of same age group differs significantly, irrespective of gender differences and chronicity of the disease'.

In order to verify the above hypothesis, 't'-test was applied for comparison of the means and standard deviations of depressive patients and normal population with regard to 'suicidal tendencies' variable as displayed in Table 4.18.

Table 4.18 shows that 't'-value is significant (p<. 01) and therefore the tenth hypothesis i.e., 'suicidal tendencies of depressive patients and normal population of same age group differs significantly, irrespective of gender differences' has been retained, which indicates that depressive patients possessed more suicidal thoughts as compared to normal counterparts.

Table 4.18: Comparison of Suicidal Tendencies of Depressive Patients and Normal Population

Sample Group	*Number*	*Mean*	*S.D.*	*'t' Value*	*Level of Signi-ficance*
Depressive Patients	118	33.89	6.88	7.15	P<. 01
Normal Population	118	39.57	6.16		

For verification of eleventh hypothesis as given below, the data were processed accordingly and is presented in Table 4.19.

'Suicidal tendencies of male and female depressive patients differ significantly, irrespective of age or chronicity of the disease'.

To check the above hypothesis, 't'-test was applied for comparing the means and standard deviations of the male and female depressive patients with regard to 'suicidal tendencies' variable as displayed in Table 4.19.

Table 4.19: Comparison of Suicidal Tendencies of Male and Female Depressive Patients

Sample Group	*Number*	*Mean*	*S.D.*	*'t' Value*	*Level of Signi-ficance*
Male Depressive Patients	63	34.82	6.86	1.62	p> .05
Female Depressive Patients	55	32.83	6.82		

From Table 4.19, it has been observed that 't' value is insignificant at .05 level (p>.05). Therefore, the eleventh hypothesis i.e., 'suicidal tendencies of male and female depressive patients differ significantly, irrespective of age or chronicity of the disease' is rejected. However, from the mean scores it can be stated that male depressive patients have lesser suicidal thoughts than the female depressive patients.

For verification of twelfth hypothesis as given below, the data were processed accordingly and is presented in Table 4.20.

'Suicidal tendencies of depressive patients differ significantly across chronicity of the disease, irrespective of gender'.

To check the above hypothesis, 't'-test was applied for comparing the means and standard deviations of the depressive patients who were suffering from depression for the last one year and more than one year as displayed in Table 4.20.

It has been observed that the patients who are suffering from depression for last one year have lesser suicidal thoughts than those of depressive patients who are suffering from depression for more than one year (p< .01). Hence, the last hypothesis i.e., 'suicidal tendencies of depressive patients differ significantly across chronicity of the disease, irrespective of gender differences' has been accepted.

Table 4.20: Comparison of Suicidal Tendencies of Depressive Patients Suffering from this Mental Health Problem for the Last One Year and More Than One Year

Depressive Patients Suffering From This Mental Health for the Last	*Number*	*Mean*	*S.D.*	*'t' Value*	*Level of Signi-ficance*
One Year	48	38.12	5.40	4.45	p< .01
More than One Year	70	31.14	6.33		

Section III: Health Seeking Behaviour, Perceived Problems and Solutions

The symptoms, which were observed in depressive patients as stated by the patient parties are provided in Table 4.21. The most common symptoms of depression as noticed among the patients include decreased energy, fatigue, being 'slowed down' (80.5%), loss of interest or pleasure in hobbies and activities that were once enjoyed, including sex (73.7%), feeling of hopelessness/pessimism (72.9%), insomnia, early morning awakening or oversleeping (66.9%), persistent sadness anxiety, anxious or 'empty mood' (66.1%), appetite and/or weight loss or overeating and weight gain (56.8%), low self-esteem (39.0%), difficulty in concentration, remembering and making decisions (34.7%), feeling of guilt, worthlessness, helplessness (29.7%), thought of death or suicide, suicidal attempts (23.7%) and others (Table 4.21).

Table 4.21: Symptoms of Depression Noticed Among Patients by the Family Members (Multiple Response)

Symptoms of Depression Noticed	*Mode of Response*	
	Frequency	*Percentage*
• Persistent sadness anxiety, anxious or 'empty mood'	78	66.1
• Feeling of hopelessness, pessimism	86	72.9
• Feeling of guilt, worthlessness, helplessness	35	29.7
• Loss of interest or pleasure in hobbies and activities that were once enjoyed, including sex	87	73.7
• Decreased energy, fatigue, being 'slowed down'	95	80.5
• Difficulty in concentrating, remembering and making decisions	41	34.7
• Insomnia, early morning awakening or oversleeping	79	66.9
• Appetite and/or weight loss or overeating and weight gain	67	56.8
• Thought of death or suicide, suicidal attempts	28	23.7
• Restlessness, irritability	15	12.7
• Low self-esteem	46	39.0
• Others like persistent physical symptoms that do not respond to treatment such as head-ache, digestive disorders and chromic pain	25	21.2

Base: All Respondents.

From Table 4.22, it is clear that there is a lack of awareness about mental health problems in our society. Only about one-fourth (23.7%) patient parties immediately consulted health service providers for advice and medication while the rest three-fourth did not pay attention to the problems of depressive patients and/or could not understand the problems.

Table 4.22: Health Seeking Behaviour

Health Seeking Behaviour	*Mode of Response*	
	Frequency	*Percentage*
• Immediately consulted doctor/ psychiatrist/psychologist	28	23.7
• Did not pay attention initial 4/6 months	49	41.5
• Patient visited doctor on his/her own	5	4.2
• First did not understand the problem, when understood visited the doctor	36	30.5

Base: All Respondents.

Causes of depression of the sample covered in the study are different as perceived by the family members. The most common cause of depression include family disturbances (56.8%), followed by prolonged health problem (18.6%), broken of marriage/affairs/long separation (16.1%), loss of close relative (15.3%), financial crisis in the family (15.1%), prolonged unemployment (13.6%), adjustment problem/poor interpersonal relationship (8.5%), and others like lose of job, work pressure, monotonous job, no issue etc. (Table 4.23).

Replying to a question what sorts of problems family members encounter in dealing with depressive patients, majority of the family members stated that withdrawn (63.6%), followed by lack of sense of responsibility (60.2%), lack of social support (57.6%), poor interpersonal relationship of the patient (57.6%), poor hygienic sense (46.6%), lack of interest in work (35.6%), irritating nature (29.7%), not attending office or work place (27.1%), suicidal attempts (23.7%), sleeping for a longer time (23.7%). Family members of the depressive patients also reported some other problems like crying, persistent physical problem; not responding to stimulus etc. (Table 4.24).

Table 4.23: Causes of Depression as Perceived by the Family Members (Multiple Response)

Perceived Causes of Depression	*Mode of Response*	
	Frequency	*Percentage*
• Poor interpersonal relationship	10	8.5
• Prolonged unemployment	16	13.6
• Family disturbances	67	56.8
• No issue/child	7	5.9
• Lose of close relative	18	15.3
• Broken of marriage/long separation/affairs	19	16.1
• Acute financial crisis in the family	18	15.1
• Loss of job	8	6.8
• Prolonged health problem	22	18.6
• Lack of achievement in life/monotonous job	6	5.1
• Prolonged health problem of the family members	8	6.8
• Others like accident, work pressure, environmental change etc.	15	12.7
• Cannot say	12	10.2

Base: All Respondents.

Table 4.24: Perceived Problems of Family Member in dealing with Depressive Patients (Multiple Response)

Perceived Problems of Family Member	*Mode of Response*	
	Frequency	*Percentage*
• Poor interpersonal relationship	68	57.6
• Poor hygienic sense/cleanliness	55	46.6
• Lack of sense of responsibility	71	60.2
• Not attending office	32	27.1
• Withdrawal	75	63.6
• Lack of interest/motivation in work	42	35.6
• Suicidal attempts	28	23.7
• Persistent physical problem	18	15.3
• Crying	22	18.6
• Irritating nature/short temperament	35	29.7
• Less social support/less support from relatives and peer group members	68	57.6
• Sleeping almost all the time	28	23.7
• Others like unable to remember, do not respond to stimulus etc.	14	18.9

Base: All Respondents.

Table 4.25: Coping Strategies of the Family Members in dealing with the Depressive Patients (Multiple Response)

Coping Strategies	*Mode of Response*	
	Frequency	*Percentage*
• Fulfilled the demand of the patients to the extent possible	35	29.7
• Provided full mental support	42	35.6
• Spent more time with the patient and listened to his/her problems patiently	25	21.2
• Never asked patient to do anything which he/she does not like	35	29.7
• Sometimes did not pay attention to his/her complaints	24	20.3
• Tried to adjust with the irritating nature of the patient	38	32.2
• Did extend full cooperation to the patient as and when required	43	36.4
• Did extend mental support to the patient to overcome his/her frustration	23	19.5
• Always helped patient in household activities	35	29.7
• Looked after the patient properly	42	35.6
• Tried to make the patient happy	35	29.7
• Tried to involve the patient in those activities which he/she used to love to do earlier	43	36.4
• Provide medicine timely to the patient as prescribed by the doctor	35	29.7
• Made every effort to over come the guilt feeling of the patient	20	16.9
• Motivated the patient that he/she is capable to come out from the depressed mood	18	15.3
• Tried to make the patient understand that we are all with his/her to overcome any problem	25	21.2
• Sometimes we become angry so that patient stops crying	27	22.8
• Tried to involve the patient in interesting activities like watching TV, indoor games, travelling, shopping, cooking, chatting etc.	38	32.2
• Followed all the instructions of doctors religiously	37	31.4
• Consulted psychiatrist immediately when situation was out of control	18	15.3
• Others like called people with whom patients relation was good, stopped interaction with the patients for a short while to make him/her understand our feeling	12	10.2

Base: All Respondents.

In order to cope with the difficult situation the patient parties adopted different strategies, which are given in Table 4.25.

Out of a total of 118 depressive patients covered in the study 28 (23.7%) attempted to commit suicide at least once. Further probing revealed that 8 attempted to commit suicide more than once (Table 4.26).

Table 4.26: History of Suicidal Attempts by Patients

Whether Attempted to Commit Suicide (Fig.9)	*Mode of Response*	
	Frequency	*Percentage*
• Yes	28	23.7
• No	90	76.3

Base: All Respondents.

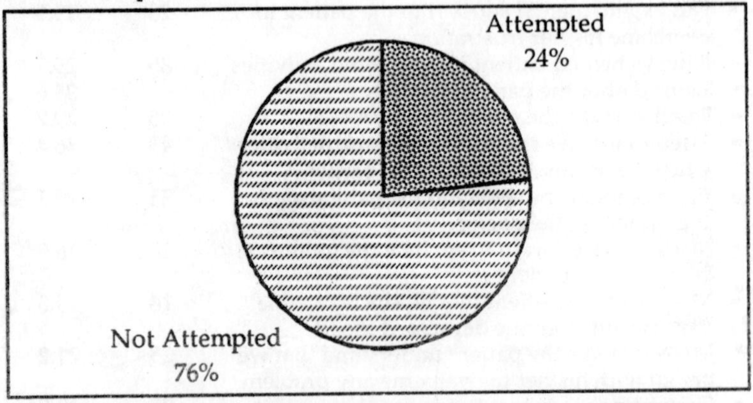

Fig. 4.9: History of Suicidal Attempts by Depressive Patients

Further, the family members of depressive patients were asked to suggest measures to deal with depressive patients more effectively on the basis of their experience. They have suggested a number of measures, which are provided in Table 4.27.

The most common measures suggested by them include providing more love and affection and mental and social support to the patients so that they feel that the family members accept them. They also asked for proper treatment of the patient including counseling by the trained counselor and medicine at affordable cost. There is a need of awareness of mental health problems among the patients parties as well as among general population is another important issue raised by the patient parties (Table 4.27).

Table 4.27: Suggested Measures to deal with Depressive Patients More Effectively—as Prescribed by the Family Members (Multiple Response)

Suggested Measures	*Mode of Response*	
	Frequency	*Percentage*
• Extend more love and affection	87	73.7
• Extend more mental support	68	57.6
• Extend more social support	79	66.9
• Extend more cooperation and adjust with the patient	78	66.1
• Need proper treatment	65	55.1
• Need regular counseling facility by a trained counselor	43	36.4
• Medicine should be available	25	21.2
• Treatment/medicine should be affordable	37	31.4
• Patient should not be blamed for his/her mental disposition	27	22.9
• Need to provide more knowledge among the patient parties about mental diseases especially about depression	26	22.0
• Require support of co-workers in the working place	17	14.4
• Doctors should listen to the problems of patient parties more carefully	38	32.2
• Govt. should arrange treatment facilities for the poor people free of cost	23	19.5
• Need to spend more time with the patient and listen to their problems	41	34.7
• Involve patients in those activities (positive) which he/she likes most	38	32.2
• Follow doctors advice properly	25	21.2
• Others like take patient out for a change, take patient in different social occasions, develop a daily activity routine for the patient and follow it up etc.	27	22.9

Base: All Respondents.

5

Discussion, Conclusion and Recommendations

Every human being in life goes through some ups and downs, and occasional sadness in life that is a normal emotion. But depression is more than feeling blue, sad, or down in the dumps once in a while. Depression is a strong mood involving sadness, discouragement, despair, or hopelessness that lasts for weeks, months, or even longer, and interferes with a person's ability to participate in their normal activities.

Depression is one of the major mental health disorders affecting a large number of population especially younger generations across the world. Currently in the United States one in every three persons is a victim of depression owing to various socio-economic, familial, psychological and environmental factors (Nelson, 1982; Andrews and Brown, 1988; Kobak et al., 1991). In India, it has affected a large number of population mainly because of unemployment, poverty, adjustment problems, loss of close family members, disturbed family relationships, stress in daily life and chronic health problems.

Depression is a common feature in case of all mental as well as physical health problems. It is very difficult to find a person who has not undergone depression once or twice in lifetime on account of different reasons. When this mental health problem affects a person for a longer time it requires medication. During this period they exhibit different problems and sometimes it becomes very difficult for the family members to deal with the patients. The family members become totally confused about the mode of treatment if the patient do not respond to some medication whether psychological or psychiatric. It happens mostly because of lack of knowledge about this mental health problem among the general population and lack of early intervention facilities in Indian society. In India normally family members do not feel like consulting a mental health professional in case of any mental health problem suffered by any one of the family members owing to social stigma. Family members consult a mental health professional as and when it becomes very difficult to manage the patient at home.

Given this background the necessity was felt to understand the mental health profile of the depressive patient in Kolkata and the types of problems encountered by the family members so that need-based measures can be suggested to deal with the problem professionally. Simultaneously literature review also indicates that no such study was carried out in India to explore the issues, which are addressed in this study.

The broad objective of the study was to ascertain the personality disposition, self-esteem, emotional control and suicidal tendencies of depressive patients. In addition, the present study also made an attempt to understand the problems encountered by the family members in dealing with depressive patients and solutions thereof. A group of 118 depressive patients, irrespective of categories were selected following incidental sampling method from different govt. and private health centres. For comparison of the data of depressive patients with regard to the variables mentioned above, a group of 118 normal population was selected purposively and they were matched in terms of age and gender. Data were collected using Bengali version of Multi-dimensional Personality Inventory by Km. Manju Agarwal, Self-esteem Inventory by M.S.Prasad and G.P.Thakur, Emotional Control Inventory by Samuel E. Krug, Suicidal Tendencies Inventory by Samuel E. Krug after local adaptation. In addition, one semi-structured questionnaires was developed by the authors and was used to gather information about socio-economic and familial background of the depressive patients. In addition, the said schedule also gathered information about the onset of the disease and the problems encountered by the family members in dealing with the patients and their suggestions thereof to deal with depressive patients more effectively. Ethical issues like informed consent, voluntary participation, confidentiality of information and convenience of data collection were taken care of while collecting data from the subjects and their family members.

Profile of the Depressive Patients

Findings revealed that the depressive patients came from all age groups. However, it mostly affected the people over 20 years of age. Out of a total of 118 depressive patients, 63 (53.4%) were male while the rest 55 (46.6%) were female which is contrary to the previous study findings (Coryell et al., 1991; Blazer et al., 1994). This could be because of gender discrimination in India. In India, males always receive better attention and care in case of health, education and food intake especially in the middle and lower socio-economic classes. In case of depression, male patients were reported more, perhaps because of their economic contribution in the family and/or for being the sole earning member in the family.

Educational background of the depressive patients indicate that it mostly affects the under graduates. Hence, it may be stated that people who could not complete graduation were unable to get better source of earning and thereby indirectly it became a cause of depression. However, people with better educational background i.e., Graduate and Post Graduate are also the victim of depression although their number is less compared to people with less education. So far as professional background is concerned, male members with both service and business background are the victims of depression. Male members who are in service are more prone to depression which could be because of work pressure, lack of future growth, unsatisfactory salary and poor interpersonal relationships. Too much competition and loss in business could be other factors for the people who suffer from depression. Interestingly, the women who are not employed i.e., the housewives become more depressed as compared to women who are employed.

So far as marital status is concerned, people of all categories become the victim of depression as 38.1% married, 23.7% single, 16.9 divorcee/separated and 21.2% widowed were found to be depressed. About two-fifth i.e., 40.7% of the patients have been suffering from depression for the last one year while the rest three-fifth (59.3%) have been suffering from the same mental health problem for more than last one year. Marital problems have also positive correlation with depression. Studies of marital couples in which one is clinically depressed have shown relatively negative interaction patterns marked by hostility, tension, difficulty resolving conflict, and reports of marital difficulties associated with depression (Gotlib and Whiffen, 1989; Gotlib and Hammen, 1992).

In Kolkata more than half of the depressive patients suffer from Dysthymic Depression (59.3%). The reason behind this could be because of stress in daily social life and poor interpersonal relationships. It is unfortunate that about one-fifth of the depressive patients did not receive any medication for a long time on account of lack of knowledge of the family members about the disease, lack of available information about the mental health services and ignorance of the family members because of poor economic condition. However, the patients who received some sorts of medication, 26.3% reported that they have fully benefited by the same while 34.7% stated that they have been benefited partially and the rest 30.5% stated that they are not at all benefited.

Family Profile of the Depressive Patients

Both psychodynamic and social learning theory models of human development emphasizes the importance of experiences in early childhood in the family environment. When those experiences are dysfunctional or when the child lacks critical experiences such as a close bond with a stable caretaker, he or she may develop maladaptive ways. Both of these models hypotheses that depression might be a form of psychopathology resulting from certain unique family experiences.

In the present study, family environment is found to have some positive link with depression since more than 70.0% patients come from disturbed family environment. A number of previous studies have also confirmed the hypothesis of disrupted family environments and relatively dysfunctional relationships between parents and children (Kaslow et al., 1994; Hammen and Rudolph, 1996). The quality of parent-child relationships is frequently impaired for depressed children. Both clinical and community samples of depressed youngsters report relatively negative interactions with their parents (Garrison et al., 1990; Cole and McPherson, 1993).

No such link of family history of depression have been found out as only 21.2% of the depressive patients came from a family with a family history of depression. However, a number of earlier studies indicated that the children of depressive patients appear to be in an increased risk for developing depression as well as other disorders (Weissman et al., 1987; Gotlib and Lee, 1990). So far as family type and size is concerned, an overwhelming number of depressive patients came from nuclear family (87.3%) with small family size.

In this regard, it is relevant to mention the notion of Bowlby (1978; 1981) with regard to depression. John Bowlby had articulated a model of the importance of early attachment bonds between the infant and caretaker, which has implications not only for depression, but also for key elements of individual personality and adaptive functioning. Specifically, Bowlby argued that infants have an innate and fundamental tendency to form attachments bonds to a primary caretaker, in the service of protection and survival. Further, the development of a stable and secure attachment bond is essential for healthy development. An infant with a mother who is consistently responsive, accessible and supportive will acquire a 'working model' i.e., cognitive representations of the self that is positive. The child will be able to use the relationship as a 'secure base' from which to explore the environment and acquire essential skills, and will form representations (beliefs and expectations) of other people as trustworthy and dependable. If, however, the attachment bond is insecure due to actual disruption or loss, or to maternal rejection, unresponsiveness, or inconsistency, the person becomes vulnerable to depression. The individual acquires negative cognitions about the self and others.

Simultaneously, poor social network is found to have positive correlation with depression. Findings of a previous study stated that depressed children report less social support, perhaps because of low social network, potentially exacerbating the ill effects of stressful family life (Daniels and Moos, 1990). A large-scale sample of medical and psychiatric patients decreased over a 2-year period as a function of availability of perceived support, and that if support was available, patients were less likely to develop a new episode (Sherbourne et al., 1995). Several studies reported that when a major life event occurs, persons who lack a supportive intimate relationship with another person are significantly more likely to develop depression (Brown and Harris, 1978; Costello, 1982).

Mental Dispositions

In the present research four metal variables of depressive patients have been studied. These are: personality dispositions, self-esteem, emotional control and suicidal tendencies.

The term 'personality' refers to the total functioning of an individual who interacts with his environment. So far as *personality disposition* is concerned, findings revealed that depressive patients and normal population differed significantly in case of all the personality variables, i.e. introversion/extroversion, self-concept, independence/dependence, temperament, adjustment and anxiety.

Introversion/extroversion has been considered as one of the important potential personality variable. Introversion—the preference for solitary activities and discomfort in social situations—is consistently associated with depression both during the episode and in remission (Hirschfeld et al., 1983; Barnett and Gotlib, 1988). Introverted behaviours and cognitions imply that a person have difficulties in their interpersonal relationships, perhaps experience less enjoyment of social situations and relationships and have less self-confidence in social occasions. Findings of the present study revealed that depressive patients and normal population differed significantly in case of introversion/extroversion variable which means that depressive patients are more introvert in nature and they act according to their own expectation and thinking.

The *self* has been considered as a central construct of the personality; the core of one's being or ego, and the end result of one's experience, the potential or the nucleus of personality. This thinking conscious entity is a complex of various vital psychological processes. It possesses a cognitive structure of adjustment and interactions. With regard to this personality variable depressive patient and normal population differed significantly which indicates that self-identification of depressive patients with a cluster of values or traits and consistency of functional existence is lower as compared to normal population.

Dependence/independence is another important variable of personality, which has close association with intelligence or uniqueness of the personality. Significant difference between depressive patients and normal population means that intellectual functioning of depressive patients is impaired as compared to normal population.

Clinical lore and empirical observations have noted that an important predictor of depression is dependency—emotional reliance on others, the belief that the affection, acceptance, and support of other people is essential to personal worth. There are two versions of this approach—one emphasizing trait dependency as a vulnerability factor, and the other emphasizing on the diathesis-stress model that depression occurs when a match between interpersonal stressors and underlying dependency motives and cognitions occurs.

The trait approach has been supported by studies showing that depressed people are relatively more dependent, even when the person is not symptomatic (Hirschfeld et al., 1986). Higher levels of dependency traits during the depressive episode may predict less likelihood of or slower recovery (Klein et al., 1988).

Temperament refers to reaction of the person toward emotional situation. By knowing about the temperament of the person one can estimate personality of the person because this is related to the consistency or mental imbalance and considered as one of the important factors of personality. Depressive patients and normal population differed significantly in temperament variable, which means that depressive patients are less consistent than those of their normal counterparts.

Adjustment is an index of integration between needs and press, which has a close relation to personality. It has been considered as a trait of personality. Significant difference between depressive patients and normal population in adjustment variable of personality means depressive patients are less capable to shape and reshape his/her personality to adjust with the changing situation in daily life.

Anxiety is generally defined as the feeling of apprehension caused by anticipation of danger, which may be internal or external. It is considered as an important personality variable. The current complexity of civilization, the rapidity of change, and the loss of certain traditional religious and familial values are creating more conflicts and anxiety in an individual's life. Present findings revealed significant difference between depressive patients and normal population in respect of anxiety variable, which indicates that depressive patients are more anxious than the non-depressed persons.

The male and female depressive patients irrespective of age or chronicity of the disease differ significantly only in case of temperament and adjustment variable. They did not differ significantly in case of rest of the personality variables, viz., extroversion/introversion, self-concept, independence/dependence and anxiety. However, mean scores indicated that male depressive patients possessed high self-concept, they were more adjusted, more independent as well as more anxious than their counterparts while female depressive patients were more introvert and short tempered as compared to their male counterparts.

Personality dispositions of depressive patients with respect to extroversion/introversion, self-concept, independence/dependence, temperament, adjustment and anxiety across chronicity of the disease differ significantly. Hence, it may be inferred that that the depressive patients who suffer from depression for more than one year are more introvert, more dependent on others, well tempered, poorly adjusted and have low anxiety along with low self-concept.

So far as *self-esteem* is concerned, it has been observed that depressive patients and normal population of same age group differed significantly which means that the self-esteem of depressive patients is low as compared to normal population. Further, findings revealed that self-esteem of male and female depressive patients irrespective of age or chronicity of the disease differed significantly, which indicates that male depressive patients possessed high self-esteem than those of female depressive patients. It could be because of outdoor activities and/or more interaction of male depressive patients with the larger society as compared to female depressive patients. Self-esteem of depressive patients across chronicity of the disease also differed significantly. From the mean score it is evident that individuals who were suffering from depression for more than one year posses low self-esteem, which means that gradually the self-esteem of depressive patients goes down.

Depression is one of several disorders generically called affective disorders, which means depression badly affects the emotion of an individual. Findings of the present study revealed that emotional control of depressive patients and normal population of same age group differed significantly which indicates that the stress tolerance level of depressive patients is low as compared to normal population. Emotional control of male and female depressive patients irrespective of age also differed significantly in the present study, which indicates that stress tolerance level of male depressive patient is higher as compared to their counterparts. In the present study, emotional control of depressive patients across chronicity of the disease also differed significantly, which means that with the passage of time the stress tolerance level of depressive patients goes down.

Some have called depression a disorder of thinking, as much as it is a disorder of mood. Depressed people typically have negative thoughts about themselves, their worlds, and the future. They experience themselves as incompetent, worthless, and are relentlessly critical of their own acts and characteristics, and often feel guilty as they dwell on their perceived shortcomings.

The cognitive features of depression have been given particular emphasis by some investigators, who note that thinking in such grim and self-critical ways actually makes people more depressed or prolongs their depression. The negativistic thinking is commonly irrational and distorted, and represents very different interpretations of the self and the world during the depressed state than an individual would typically display when they weren't depressed. This observation gave rise to Aaron Beck's cognitive model of depression (Beck, 1967). Findings of the present study reveal that suicidal thoughts of depressive patients and normal population of same age group differed significantly which indicates that depressive patients have lost hope in life and wish to end their lives.

One of the most noteworthy characteristics of depression is that it is far more common among women than men (Weissman and Olfson, 1995). This apart, there are also indications that the women's course of depression is different from men's. For example, women may have earlier onsets than men do (Sorenson, Rutter and Aneshensel, 1991). However in the present study male and female depressive patients did not differ significantly with regard to suicidal tendencies variable. Suicidal tendencies of depressive patients across chronicity of the disease differ significantly. Interestingly, the people who are suffering from depression for more than last one year possess more suicidal thoughts as compared to the depressive patients who are suffering from depression for the last one year.

In India, general population and even the educated people neither have adequate knowledge about mental health problems nor they are aware of services available for the same. Findings of the present study corroborate the said above statement since only about one-fourth (23.7%) patient parties immediately consulted health service providers for advice and medication while the rest of the three-fourth did not pay attention to the problems of depressive patients and/or could not understand the problems. The issue requires attention of health policy-makers for the needful steps.

Whenever there is a patient in the family with mental health problem, in reality all the family members become victim of anxiety, stress and depression, thinking about the remedy of the said mental patient in the family. It also affects the output of the entire individual in the family, as they remain busy with the patients. Hence it is loss of human resource. In order to understand the problems faced by the family members in dealing with a depressive patients, it has been observed that majority of the family members stated that withdrawal (63.6%) is the common problem of depressive patients, followed by lack of sense of responsibility (60.2%), lack of social support (57.6%), poor interpersonal relationship of the patient (57.6%), poor hygienic sense (46.6%), lack of interest in work (35.6%), irritating nature (29.7%), not attending office or work place (27.1%), suicidal attempts (23.7%), sleeping for a longer time (23.7%), crying (18.6%), and others like unable to remember, not responding to stimulus (18.9%) (Chapter IV, Table 4.24).

Out of a total of 118 depressive patients covered in the present study 23.7% attempted to commit suicide at least once. Further probing revealed that 8 attempted to commit suicide more than once. Greenberg (1982) reported that as many as half of the suicides in the United States are committed by people suffering from depression. Suicidal ideation is quite common in depressed youngsters (Mitchell et al., 1988; Ryan et al., 1987). Actual suicidal attempts occurred in 39.0% of the preadolescents and adolescent samples of Mitchell et al., (1988), with 6.0-12.0% of the Ryan et al., (1987) child and adolescent samples making moderate or severe attempts. These rates appear to be higher among depressed youngsters than among depressed adults.

Direct and/or first hand experienced people are the right kind of persons to suggest the remedial measures after the specialized professionals. In the present study, effort was made to understand the viewpoints of first-hand experienced people about the remedy to deal with depressive patients. They have suggested a number of measures. The most common measures as suggested by the family members include providing more love and affection, mental and social support to the patients so that they feel that they are accepted to the family members. They also asked for proper treatment of the patients including counseling by the trained counselor and medicine at affordable cost and/or free of cost. There is also a need for awareness of mental health problems among the patient's parties as well as among general population as suggested by the family members.

Conclusion

In fine, it may be stated that depressive patients differ significantly with their normal counterparts with regard to mental health variables like personality dispositions, self-esteem, emotional control and suicidal tendencies.

Further, gender-wise significant difference was observed in case of self-esteem and emotional control of depressive patients while no significant difference was observed with regard to suicidal tendencies. However, in case of personality variables male and female depressive patients differed significantly only with regard to temperament and adjustment variables.

Findings also revealed that in case of all the mental health variables i.e., personality dispositions, self-esteem, emotional control and suicidal tendencies, depressive patients differ significantly across chronicity of the disease, irrespective of gender differences.

Findings of the present study revealed the general population lack awareness about the mental health problems and there is shortage of professional services for the mentally disturbed people in our society. Findings also unearthed the type of problems encountered by the patient parities in dealing with depressive patients and explored the suggestions as to how to deal with depressive patients more effectively.

Recommendations for Future Study

On the basis of the findings of the present study, the following studies are recommended for future researchers:

- One study should be carried out to understand the level of stress among general population across different social strata.
- Another study should be carried out to unearth whether mental depression is most responsible for family disturbances or vice versa.
- Further, it would be very helpful if evaluation of different psychological intervention programmes for prognosis of depression are carried out to understand the efficacy of the same so that professionals can follow the most effective intervention programme.

Recommendations for Diagnosis of the Disease and Intervention

On the basis of the findings of the present study and keeping the fact in mind that depression is the most common prevalent feature among all the mental health problems, the following steps have been recommended.

- There should be proper arrangements of psychodiagnosis in the Govt. and Non-Govt. hospitals for ascertaining the mental state especially about suicidal thoughts among the depressive patients. So that timely intervention can be provided to the needy patients.
- Complete case history and psychiatric interview should be taken along with physical examination to determine if the cause of depression is physical or psychological.
- Proper mental status examination should be carried out by the trained Psychologist emphasizing on current

stressors, support system, dependence on substances and suicidal ideation.

- The doctor may recommend medication, but treatment will vary according to the cause and severity of the depressive symptoms, as well as patient's preference. If patient is undergoing any other medications that could cause depression, these may need to be changed. Medications should not be changed without consulting the health-care provider.
- For mild depressive symptoms, counseling from experienced counseller may be recommended.
- For moderate to severe depression, anti-depressant medication may be prescribed. Psychotherapy may also be recommended. Several types of focused psychotherapies have been developed that are as effective as medication in treating depression. The choice of medications, psychotherapy, or both can be made based on patient's preference and the availability of these treatments. In order to avoid recurrent bouts of depression, it is important to finish the course of treatment.
- For people who are severely depressed as to be unable to function, or who are so acutely suicidal they cannot be safely cared for in the community, psychiatric hospitalization may be necessary.
- More mental support should be provided to the depressive patients in the home set up. For the said purpose there should be some arrangements for orientation of the family members in the Govt. and Non-Govt. hospitals so that the family members can deal with the depressive patients more effectively.
- For mild depressive symptoms, improving health habits to provide adequate and regular sleep and good nutrition may bring relief. Regular exercise is also helpful. Decreasing the use of alcohol and other drugs is also recommended, since these can aggravate depressive symptoms.

- Involvement in healthy pleasures such as recreation and creative activities, and staying involved with family and friends helps to lift a person's mood.
- Being reminded that other people's care helps to relieve the isolation that often accompanies depressed feelings. Discussion with clergy or spiritual advisers may give meaning to painful experiences, and prayer or meditation can access internal sources of strength.
- If you recognize that your family member who is suffering from depression is chronically pessimistic and self-critical, self-help workbooks to combat depressive thinking may be helpful. These usually involve a programme of exercises to identify distorted perceptions and substitute more realistic ones. But when you or a loved one cannot shake these feelings within a few weeks or with help from sources above mentioned, you may need to contact your doctor, because you may be suffering from major depression.
- Depression disrupts work and family life for more than two weeks. Depression is so severe that suicide is contemplated. Do not hesitate to call for help immediately, if your primary health-care provider can't be reached, many communities have telephone hotlines for such situations. If there is no such service nearby, call the nearest emergency room or health-care facility.
- Professional mental health services should be made available for the mentally disturbed individuals in all the Govt. and Non-Govt. hospitals and it should be a part of regular health services since in our country the incidence of various types of mental problem is increasing steadily.
- Social support system should be improved i.e., the depressive patients should be taken to different social occasions and should be allowed to take part in daily life activities under proper supervision.
- Arrangements of free treatment facilities should be made available in the Govt. Health Centres including free medicines for the poor people.

- There should be proper referral services in the Govt. and Non-Govt. hospitals i.e., the list of local psychiatrists, psychologists, family counselors, and rehabilitation homes for mentally disturbed people and list of emergency services should be available. This referral services will benefit the patient parties as and when required.
- Anti-depressant medications are widely used, effective treatments for depression. Existing anti-depressants influence the functioning of certain chemicals in the brain called neurotransmitters. The newer medications, such as the selective serotonin reuptake inhibitors (SSRIs), tend to have fewer side effects than the older drugs, which include tricyclic anti-depressants (TCAs) and monoamine oxidase inhibitors (MAOIs). Although both generations of medications are effective in relieving depression, some people will respond to one type of drug, but not another. Other types of anti-depressants are now in development.
- Certain types of psychotherapy, specifically cognitive-behavioural therapy (CBT) and interpersonal therapy (IPT), have been found helpful for depression. Research indicates that mild to moderate depression often can be treated successfully with either therapy alone; however, severe depression appears more likely to respond to a combination of psychotherapy and medication. More than 80 per cent of people with depressive disorders improve when they receive appropriate treatment (*Source*: National Institute of Mental Health, 2002).
- Treatment for Dysthymia Disorder consists of a combination of medication and therapy. The most common therapies are cognitive therapy and behavioural therapy. Often, higher doses of medications are necessary than for severe depression.
- Workshops and seminars should be organized to create awareness among general population about causes and consequences of various mental health problems with

a view to eradicating the superstition and social stigma about the mental health problems.

The Art of Avoiding Depression

In every sense, depression is a growing problem. Rates of depression have steadily climbed over the last 50 years and are significantly higher in those born after 1945 than in those born before. In addition, the average age of onset of a first depressive episode is steadily decreasing—it is now mid-20s whereas it once was mid-30s. Cross-cultural data show that the United States has a higher rate of depression than almost any other country, and that as Asian countries Westernize their rates of depression increase correspondingly.

The data make it abundantly clear that these changes are not the product of individual biochemistry or of family genetics but of pathology within our culture. There are many depressogenic factors operating in our culture. Information overload is one. Since 1945 we have accumulated at least as much information as we had throughout history until then. The more information there is, the more we end up essentially skimming the surface. This leads to a style of thinking in which we see only the big picture and miss the details. As a result, when we are faced with difficult problems, we do not recognize the many small steps that solutions typically require; things feel overwhelming and insurmountable, leading us to give up before we even start.

Our growing reliance on technology also contributes to depression. One of technology's main values is speed. But speed has altered our perspective of time so that we expect things to happen at ever-faster rates. Embracing speed as a cultural value has advantages when we are dealing with things that can actually be done quickly, such as electronic mail, but it is a profound disadvantage when applied to other domains of life, like building a relationship. We can't instantly learn to be a good judge of other people's character or instantly build good relationships with our colleagues at our new job. But people want a good relationship, and they want it now, without having a clue what the steps are and how long it takes to achieve each one. They expect instant intimacy and fool themselves into thinking they've achieved it by sleeping with somebody before they know who the person is.

It has become fashionable to call depression a disease, to medicalize it. And certainly neurotransmitters like serotonin and norepinephrine are involved in depression. But if we ask more critical question—is biology the cause of depression?—the best data suggest that genes account for about one in five cases. The idea that a chemical imbalance causes depression, rather than reflects it, ignores the fact that the brain's biochemistry responds to our ways of thinking—in short, to life experience.

Depression is an organized, patterned way of responding to events and experiences. For example, some people develop the tendency to take things personally, even when things are not personal or they tend to engage in all-or-nothing thinking. Either way, the result is that they draw wrong conclusions about events and make the mistake of believing those conclusions rather than testing them. A person whose relationship has broken up tells himself, "No person will ever love me, I'll never fall in love again." And he doesn't, unless somebody comes along and challenges that false belief.

It has long been assumed that when depression runs in families the cause is defective genes. But parents also transmit their general patterns of perception and thinking to their children. Some children are programmed early in life to make grossly negative interpretations about themselves. They bring home an A-minus grade and their father says, "You're a lazy kid. You're grounded until you get an A." Just like that they learn that they're nothing without the A, that it's all or nothing.

Depression is helped most when we encourage people to be active on their own behalf, to challenge their own thinking, to find out whether the thoughts that hurt them are true or not. That's why psychotherapy outperforms medication in the long run. In studies comparing drug therapy to psychotherapy for depression, after about a month medications are ahead; they provide a reduction of symptoms more quickly and more reliably than therapy does. After a couple of months, antidepressants and psychotherapy are running neck and neck; at 12 weeks, therapy is actually slightly ahead. Clients feel better about themselves when they're taking action on their own behalf and learning the principles that will help insulate them from later episodes of depression. As a result, relapse occurs 50 per cent more often among patients receiving medication alone than among those receiving both drugs and therapy.

Cognitive therapy, behavioural therapy, interpersonal therapy, and medication all work. But, no matter what, you do need a variety of skills in order to avoid depression. Here are some of them:

- Perhaps the most important skill is the ability to recognize and tolerate ambiguity. In many situations there is no single correct answer but a variety of possibilities. Life is inherently ambiguous; an experiential Rorschach. It is in response to ambiguity that we're most likely to make the negative interpretations that can lead to depression.
- Critical thinking is crucial for overcoming depression. It means the ability to examine the evidence and correctly assess the truth of our beliefs, to discriminate between things that we're responsible for and things that we're not. People tend to underestimate or overestimate the amount of control they actually have over situations. If they assume they're helpless when they're not, they don't even try. The ability to recognize what you are and are not responsible for is directly related to how much guilt you experience.
- You need to discriminate between ways in which you are defined by your achievements and ways that you are not. Times when it's okay to get in touch with your feelings, and those when you'd better get out of touch with them, when it's okay to focus on the present, and when it's better to concentrate on the future.
- Another crucial skill is the ability to clearly articulate goals. Wanting to be happy is not an unreasonable goal.

But what exactly do you mean by 'happy'? You should know your goal and you should have proper planning for achieving the goal.

- A highly important skill for warding off depression is learning to discriminate between what you feel versus what is objectively true. Good mental health requires you to juggle the interplay between what's going on within you and what is going on out there.
- Finally, relationship skills are important for preventing depression. We've known for decades that relationships serve as buffers against illness and emotional disorders. The people who are at the greatest risk for depression are those who are most lonely. Demographically, single women face the highest risk; married men, the lowest. So it's crucial to know how to meet people, assess them, communicate with them, let them know you're interested in them. And once you're in a relationship, you need to take steps to keep it healthy, such as asserting personal boundaries and setting up the rules by which the relationship will operate (Yapko, Michael. D., 1997).

Love Needs

Love is as critical for our mind and body as oxygen. It's not negotiable. The more connected we are, the healthier we will be both physically and emotionally. The less connected we are, the more we are at risk.

It is also true that the less love we have, the more depression we are likely to experience in our life. Love is probably the best anti-depressant because one of the most common sources of depression is feeling unloved. Most depressed people don't love themselves and they do not feel loved by others. They also are very self-focused, making them less attractive to others and depriving them of opportunities to learn the skills of love.

There is a mythology in our culture that love just happens. As a result, the depressed often sit around passively waiting for someone to love them. But love doesn't work that way. To get love and keep love you have to go out and be active and learn a variety of specific skills.

Most of us get our ideas of love from popular culture. We come to believe that love is something that sweeps us off our feet. But the pop-culture ideal of love consists of unrealistic images created for entertainment, which is one reason so many of us are set up to be depressed. We think it is love when it's simply distraction and infatuation.

One consequence is that when we hit real love we become upset and disappointed because there are many things that do not fit the cultural ideal. Some of us get demanding and controlling, wanting someone else to do what we think our ideal of romance should be, without realizing our ideal is misplaced.

It is not only possible but necessary to change one's approach to love to ward off depression. Follow these action strategies to get more of what you want out of life—to love and be loved.

- Recognize the difference between limerance and love. Limerance is the psychological state of deep infatuation. It feels good but rarely lasts. Limerance is that first stage of mad attraction whereby all the hormones are flowing and things feel so right. Limerance lasts, on average, six months. It can progress to love. Most cases of love in fact starts out as limerance, but mostly limerance never evolves into love.
- Know that love is a learned skill, not something that comes from hormones or emotion particularly. Erich Fromm called it "an act of will." If you don't learn the skills of love you virtually guarantee that you will be depressed, not only because you will not be connected enough but because you will have many failure experiences.
- Learn good communication skills. They are means by which you develop trust and intensify connection. The more you can communicate the less depressed you will be because you will feel known and understood.

- Focus on the other person. Rather than focus on what you are getting and how you are being treated, read your partner's need. What does this person really need for his/her own well-being? This is a very tough skill for people to learn in our narcissistic culture. Of course, you don't lose yourself in the process; you make sure you're also doing enough self-care.
- Help someone else. Depression keeps people so focused on themselves they don't get beyond themselves enough to be able to learn to love. The more you can focus on others and learn to respond and meet their needs, the better you are going to do in love.
- Develop the ability to accommodate simultaneous reality. The loved one's reality is as important as your own, and you need to be as aware of it as of your own. What are they really saying, what are they really needing? Depressed people think the only reality is their own depressed reality.
- Actively dispute with yourself internal messages of inadequacy. Sensitivity to rejection is a cardinal feature of depression. As a consequence of low self-esteem, every relationship is interpreted far too personally as evidence of inadequacy. Quick to feel rejected by a partner, you then believe it is the treatment you fundamentally deserve. But the rejection really originates in you, and the feelings of inadequacy are the depression speaking.
- Recognize that the internal voice is strong but it's not real. Talk back to it. "I'm not really being rejected, this isn't really evidence of inadequacy. I made a mistake." Or "this isn't about me, this is something I just didn't know how to do and now I'll learn." When you reframe the situation to something more adequate, you can act again in an effective way and you can find and keep the love that you need (Ellen McGrath, 2002).

Appendix I

Date of Interview: ....

Background Information Schedule

Developed by

Dr. Sibnath Deb and Anjana Bhattacharjee
Department of Applied Psychology,
University of Calcutta
(2002)

Introduction: The broad objective of this schedule is to gather information about the socio-economic and family background of the subjects. This schedule also intends to gather information about the problems encountered by the family members in dealing with depressive patients. There are no right or wrong answers. We are interested to know your personal opinion about the following issues. Please note that confidentiality of the information will be maintained and information will be used for research purpose only. Hence, feel free to share the information.

Section I: Socio-economic and Treatment Related Information

1.1 Name of the Subject and Address, (specify Urban or Rural and congested or uncongested living environment) :...
....
....
....
....

1.2 Age:
Below 20..............................1 41-45 6
21-25 ....2 46-50 7
26-30 ....3 51-55 8
31-35 ....4 56 and above 9
36-40 5

1.3 Gender: Male ....1, Female 2

1.4 Education:
Below Madhyamik........... 1 Graduate 4
Madhyamik ....2 Post Graduate and above 5
H.S. passed 3

1.5. Occupation:
Service ....1 Unemployed 3
Student ....2 Business 4
Others, pl. specify 5

1.6 Marital Status:
Married..........................1 Divorce 3
Single/Unmarried ....2 Widow 4

1.7 Income:
Below 4000 per month 1 Rs.12001-16000 4
Rs. 4001-8000 ....2 Rs. 16001 and above
.........5
Rs. 8001-12000 3

1.8 Onset of Depression:
Up to one month............1 One to two years..............4
One to six months..........2 Two years and above 5
Six months to one year.....3

1.9 Whether treatment received:
Yes.................................1 No 2

1.10 If yes, whether benefitted:
Yes.................................1 No 2

1.11 Type of depression:
Major Depression 1
Dysthymic 2
Bipolar Depression 3

1.12 Whether the subject suffers from any major physical health problem?
Yes..................................1 No 2

1.13 If yes, what is the health problem?

____

____

1.14 For how long the subject is suffering from the same health problem:
For the last six months 1
For the last one year...................................2
For the last two years.................................3
For the last three years 4
More than three years 5

1.15 Any addiction: Yes ....1, No 2

1.16 If yes, dependent on what:
Alcohol ....1 Sleeping Tablets..................3
Drug...................................2 Others, please specify 4

1.17 No. of siblings:
One.....................................1 Three 3
Two.....................................2 Four and above 4

Section II: Family Related Information

2.1 Any family history of depression:
Yes .... 1, No 2

2.2 Type of family:
Joint ....1, Single 2

2.3 Size of family:
Below 4 members..........1 7-8 members 3
4-6 members................2 9 and above 4

2.4 Family environment:
Peaceful........................1
Not so peaceful.................2
Disturbed 3

2.5 In general subject's relation with the family members:
Very friendly 1
Not so friendly 2
Disturbed 3

2.6 Any addiction/deviant habit/background of any of the family members:
Yes ....1, No 2

2.7 If yes, please state the relationship of the said person with the subject:

2.8 Total family income from all sources:
Below Rs. 4000 ....1 Rs.12001-16000 4
per month
Rs. 4001-8000 ....2 Rs. 16001 and above 5
Rs. 8001-12000...............3

2.9 Social network of family:
Low social network 1
Moderate social network 2
High social network 3

2.10 Whether any family member is suffering from any major physical health problem?
Yes ....1, No 2

2.11 If yes, what is the health problem?

2.12 For how long he/she has been suffering from the same health problem:
For the last six months..........................1
For the last one year 2
For the last two years............................3
For the last three years............................4
More than four years...............................5

Section III: Problems Perceived by the Family Members in Dealing with Depressive Patient

3.1 When family members first noticed the problem in subject?
Six months back...............1
One-Two years back.........2
Three-Four years back......3
Five and above years........4

3.2 What were the symptoms?

Symptoms	*Code No.*
• Persistent sad, anxious or 'empty mood'	1
• Feeling of hopelessness, pessimism	2
• Feeling of guilt, worthlessness, helplessness	3
• Loss of interest or pleasure in hobbies and activities that were once enjoyed, including sex	4
• Decreased energy, fatigue, being 'slowed down'	5
• Difficulty in concentrating, remembering, making decisions	6
• Insomnia, early morning awakening, or oversleeping	7
• Appetite and/or weight loss or overeating and weight gain	8
• Thoughts of death or suicide, suicidal attempts	9
• Restlessness, irritability	10
• Low self-esteem	11
• Persistent physical symptoms that do not respond to treatment such as headache, digestive disorders and chronic pain	12
• Others, please specify	13

3.3 What did they do?
Immediately contacted doctor 1
Did not pay attention 2
Any other, please specify 3

3.4 What are the probable causes as perceived by the family members?
Poor academic performance 1
Prolonged unemployment.. 2
Family disturbances.. 3
No issue/child... 4
Lose of close relative 5
Stressful working condition 6
Others, please specify 7

3.5 What sorts of problems do they encounter in dealing with the subject? (DON'T PROMPT, PROPBE THOROUGHLY)
Poor interpersonal relationships,
specify with whom 1
Poor hygienic sense/cleanliness,
specify in regard to what 2

Lack of sense of responsibility,
specify............ 3
Not attending office..4
Withdrawn,
specify..5
Others, please specify 6

3.6 How did you deal with the situation?

____

____

____

____

____

3.7 Whether subject attempted to commit suicide?
Yes ....1, No 2

3.8 If yes, how many times?
Once 1
Twice...2
More than twice 3

3.9 According to you, what needs to be done to deal with these types of patients?

____

____

____

____

APPENDIX II

Multidimensional Personality Inventory

Developed by
Km. Manju Agarwal (1988) and locally adapted by
Anjana Bhattacharjee and Dr. Sibnath Deb (2002)

Instruction: Some statements are given here. Please go through these statements carefully. There are three possible answers i.e., 'yes', 'sometimes' and 'no' beside each statement. If you totally agree to the statement then put a tick (√) mark to the category of 'yes' and if you do not agree then put a tick (√) to 'no'. Similarly, if you fell that the statement is sometimes applicable to you, please put a tick mark (√) to 'sometimes.'

There is no right or wrong answer in this inventory. Please respond to all the items without any hesitation. There is no time limit but still try your best to complete these statements as early as you can. If you feel any difficulty, please tell me. Your responses will be kept confidential.

Name:..

Age:.. Sex:..

Education:.............................. Occupation:...........................

Address:...

....

Sl. No.	*Statements*	*Mode of Response*		
		Yes	*Some-times*	*No*
	(A)			
1.	I wish to work alone so that I can work according to myself.			
2.	A work done in Cooperation gets spoiled.			
3.	Without any reason I do not meet people.			
4.	I go with my friends in social occasions.			
5.	I feel uneasy if my friends do not seat beside me in the office or in the cinema hall.			
6.	I use to stand beside of my neighbours in both pleasures sadful situation.			
7.	I do not hesitate to highlight others faults.			
8.	I work according to myself even after knowing faults and weaknesses of others.			
9.	I have a habit to make friendship even with the strangers at a new place.			
10	Often on seeing me my friends uses to tell me that I do not take their opinions in my work.			
11.	Often I share my belongings to others.			
12.	Often I sit alone and do my study.			
13.	I prefer to study alone in a closed room while listening to music rather than studying jointly with my friends.			
14.	As I am suspicious minded, I do not have many friends.			
15.	I can easily make my work done from any strangers.			
16.	I cannot keep my secretes within myself.			
17.	I feel very happy in taking active participation in social activities.			
18.	I do not take part in pleasure—sorrow activities of the society thinking that such events happen very often in this world.			
19.	I become upset whenever any past event comes to my mind.			
20.	Whenever I travel, many travellers become my friend.			
	(B)			
1.	I think that I am an efficient person.			
2.	I wish to get respect from my friends.			
3.	I am capable of doing everything.			
4.	I think that I am very powerful.			

(contd)

(contd)

Sl. No.	*Statements*	*Mode of Response*		
		Yes	*Some-times*	*No*
5.	I have faith on ability and hard work.			
6.	I have many qualities so I can solve my problems by my own.			
7.	I work according to my own wish.			
8.	I use to think very deeply about my own problems.			
9.	People know it very well that I do have all qualities.			
10.	I can do any kind of work.			
11.	I give priority to my present rather than thinking of my future.			
12.	I do not care of others anger.			
13.	Every body praises' my work and me.			
14.	I am of stubborn nature.			
15.	My friends think that I am very proudy.			
16.	I can easily impress others by my personality.			
17.	I become very upset when I see others' sorrow.			
18.	I am efficient to solve problem.			
19.	I am very much concern about my responsibilities rather than giving priority to my rights.			
20.	I have a strong desire to become a rich person.			
	(C)			
1.	I want to do such work, which will make me self-dependent.			
2.	I use to solve my problem in such a way that I may lead a happy life.			
3.	I like such syllabus that may help me to get a job in future.			
4.	I am mature enough now so I wish to work seriously.			
5.	I don't want to be a burden on my family and society.			
6.	Everybody likes me for my work procedure.			
7.	I become very much angry if my parents interfere too much in my activities.			
8.	I do not worry of getting job because I have enough quality to get a job.			
9.	I feel that I am mentally mature.			
10.	I like to work without any help.			
11.	I like to work rather than living in fantasy.			

(contd)

(contd)

Sl. No.	*Statements*	*Mode of Response*		
		Yes	*Some-times*	*No*
12.	I believe in the theory that outcome will certainly be the result of one's own work.			
13.	I do not do any such work, which can make me frightened.			
14.	Seeing my self-dependency, people think that I will become a very rich person.			
15.	I do not like any interference in my thoughts and works.			
16.	I am not a burden on my parents.			
17.	I don't like anyone to object me while roaming with my friends.			
18.	I like to stay alone because I make most of my planning by my own.			
19.	I feel irritated, as people do not consider me as self-dependent.			
20.	My friends and my family members have faith on me.			
	(D)			
1.	My friends think of my nature as faulty.			
2.	I wish my friends didn't oppose me.			
3.	Often I face lots of problems due to my nature.			
4.	My teachers get irritated on account of my nature and behaviour.			
5.	I get angry even for silly matters.			
6	I least bother about whether my friends talk to me or not.			
7.	Due to my blunt and critical talk my friends do not behave properly with me.			
8.	People are jealous of me due to my nature.			
9.	When I see that people want me to flatter, I hate them.			
10.	I know that due to my nature I can't make many friends.			
11.	I became mentally disturbed when my family members tell me to do such work, which I don't want to do.			
12.	Often my friends take advantage of my simplicity.			
13.	Whatever people say, I don't mind.			

(contd)

(contd)

Sl. No.	Statements	Mode of Response		
		Yes	Some-times	No
14.	When I am unsuccessful, I become upset for several days.			
15.	I feel like biting my younger if they disobey me.			
16.	My behaviour changes when I find things are in disorder.			
17.	I became upset if any work is not done according to my wish.			
18.	Generally my personality is balanced.			
19.	When I get angry, I never say anything to others but I stop taking food.			
20.	I use to keep my patience in any work even if that work is against my nature.			
	(E)			
1.	I like this world.			
2.	My friends like me very much.			
3.	Being intelligent in class, my teachers consider me as good student.			
4.	I wish to have many friends & have friendly terms with them.			
5.	My friends and family members like me very much.			
6.	I think that there are many means available in this world to live a luxurious life.			
7.	When I will be grown up, I would like to work in such a way so that everybody could lead a happy and prosperous life.			
8.	My younger and elder brothers and sisters like me very much.			
9.	I am more eager to know that for which job or business I will be eligible rather than concentrating on studies.			
10.	After being educated only I will do job.			
11.	I do not bother whether friendship remains or not.			
12.	I can't control my emotions.			
13.	There is no value for a good person in this world.			
14.	My father considers my opinion in every family matters.			

(contd)

(contd)

Sl. No.	*Statements*	*Mode of Response*		
		Yes	*Some-times*	*No*
15.	Everybody is eager to make friendship with me.			
16.	I never oppose my parents.			
17.	I try to keep everybody happy.			
18.	My neighbours like me very much.			
19.	In social activities I energetically take part.			
20.	Whenever I get time, I use to help my family members in the household work.			
	(F)			
1.	Sometimes I feel to change the society.			
2.	Everybody thinks I am worthless.			
3.	I don't bother over that each individual in this world suffers from misery on account of one or the other cause.			
4.	I am free from all anxiety.			
5.	I like more sad songs.			
6.	The cause of my anxiety is the inability in studies.			
7.	I fear of failure in the examination.			
8.	My friends are jealous of me.			
9.	The world is so selfish that no one can live here with truth and honesty.			
10.	There is risk in every work.			
11.	Everyone in this world feels jealous of me and hates me.			
12.	I am anxious of getting a good job.			
13.	Nothing to worry about a job, only that will happen what is written in fate.			
14.	I worry over that everybody gets angry with me.			
15.	I am anxious of becoming self-dependent.			
16.	I am anxious of making my life prosperous.			
17.	Often I feel anxious about my general physical health.			
18.	I try to keep proper adjustment with the society.			
19.	I worry about how to make good friends.			
20.	I try to behave nicely with the family members yet they assault me even for the very minor things.			

APPENDIX III

Self-esteem Inventory

Developed By
M.S. Prasad and G.P. Thakur (1989) and locally adapted by
Anjana Bhattacharjee and Dr. Sibnath Deb (2002)

Instruction: Several questions are given in this questionnaire. You read them carefully one by one. Each question consists of seven categories of answers—'Totally Correct', 'Correct to a Large Extent', 'Partially Correct', 'Uncertain,' 'Partially Wrong', 'Wrong to a Large Extent', 'Totally Wrong'. You are expected to put a correct mark (√) in the particular category, which in your view is appropriate for you, related to the statements. While replying you have to keep this thing in mind that what the people who know you think about you. Following the same way you have to reply all the statements of the questionnaire. Please reply serially.

At the end please check that you have expressed your opinion about every statements. There is no time limit for answering but please reply as early as you can without any hesitation. Your responses will be kept confidential.

Name:..

Age:.. Sex:...

Education:.............................. Occupation:...........................

Address:..

....

Sl. No.	Statements	Mode of Response* 1	2	3	4	5	6	7
1.	I am of very kind nature.							
2.	I am of irritating nature.							
3.	Honesty is the best policy in my life.							
4.	I am not a miser but calculative.							
5.	I have the capacity to adjust with any situation.							
6.	I am obstinate by nature.							
7	I do not like to see things disturbed.							
8.	I can easily control my emotions.							
9.	I feel ashamed to learn something from my juniors.							
10.	I can't easily trust others.							
11.	I like flattering.							
12.	I do obey my duties faithfully.							
13.	I can easily influence others by my personality.							
14.	I am not a moralist, I am materialist.							
15.	I do not suffer from inferiority complex.							
16.	I do not consider myself as intelligent.							
17	I can easily make friendship with strangers.							
18.	I am quarrelsome by nature.							
19.	I do not consider anyone superior in my contemporaries.							
20.	I don't get disappointed even if I am not successful.							
21.	I like to work alone rather working jointly.							
22.	I have a habit to destroy things.							
23.	I think myself beautiful.							
24.	I consider hard work as the only key to success.							
25.	I am not able to tolerate others success.							
26.	I do consider it my duty to follow ruled and get it followed.							
27.	I don't believe in advocating.							
28.	I become very angry if anyone does not trust me.							
29.	I do not take it bad to violate the rules occasionally.							
30.	I have strong desire to become a great man.							

* *1=Totally Correct; 2=Correct to a Large Extent; 3=Partially Correct; 4=Uncertain; 5=Partially Wrong; 6= Wrong to a Large Extent; 7= Totally Wrong.*

Emotional Control Inventory

Developed by Samuel E. Krug (1989) and locally adapted by Anjana Bhattacharjee and Dr. Sibnath Deb (2002)

Instruction: Fifteen statements are given in this questionnaire. Each statement consists of three possible answers. Read each statement carefully one after another and then put a tick mark (√) to the answer, which you feel is appropriate for you.

There is no right or wrong answer in this inventory. Please respond to all the items without any hesitation. There is no time limit but still try your best to complete these as early as you can. If you feel any difficulty please tell immediately. Your responses will be kept confidential.

Name:..
Age:.. Sex:..
Education:............................... Occupation:...........................
Address:..
....

1. **I hardly get impatient and angry with people.**
   (i) Yes, I hardly do.
   (ii) Sometimes I do.
   (iii) No, I easily get impatient and angry
2. **I can keep my mind steady in doing any work or any planning.**
   (i) Yes, almost always.
   (ii) Sometimes.
   (iii) No, not very often.
3. **When others give me responsibility to complete any work by my own, I get anxious of completing it correctly.**
   (i) Yes, often I get anxious.
   (ii) Sometimes I get anxious.
   (iii) No, hardly I get anxious
4. **Any great provincial festival should be marked by grandeur and splendor.**
   (i) Yes, it should be.
   (ii) Uncertain.
   (iii) No, it should not be.
5. **If acquaintances treat me badly and show they dislike me.**
   (i) I feel depressed.
   (ii) Sometimes I feel depressed.
   (iii) I never feel so.
6. **I feel more irritated with those people who cannot tolerate others success than to those who always talk about their own problems.**
   (i) Yes, I feel irritated.
   (ii) Sometimes I feel.
   (iii) No, I never feel so.
7. **While talking I hardly walk around or use my arms to express my ideas.**
   (i) Yes, I hardly do.
   (ii) Sometimes I do.
   (iii) No, I never do.

8. **I cannot tolerate those people who shows false pride or who always try to show that they are great.**
   (i) Yes, I cannot tolerate.
   (ii) Sometimes I can.
   (iii) I can easily tolerate them.
9. **If I could get right training, I would rather be**
   (i) A manager who improves efficacy in the company.
   (ii) Uncertain
   (iii) The leader and guide of the youth.
10. **I take active participation in any social gathering.**
   (i) Yes, always I take.
   (ii) Sometimes I take
   (iii) No, hardly I take.
11. **In taking any decision I give more importance on.**
   (i) What is right or wrong?
   (ii) Sometimes-on right and sometimes on wrong.
   (iii) What is practicable and workable?
12. **To be more cautious and not expecting too much is better than to be more cheerful and always expecting success.**
   (i) I agree with this statement.
   (ii) Uncertain
   (iii) No, I don't agree.
13. **I like to be one who tells others what to do.**
   (i) Yes, I like.
   (ii) Uncertain.
   (iii) No, I don't like.
14. **If the plate is least/bit dirty, I feel too disgusted to have food on it.**
   (i) Yes, often I feel.
   (ii) Sometimes I feel.
   (iii) No, never I feel so.
15. **If I had ideas about novel kitchen appliances for facilitating kitchen job.**
   (i) I would have experimented with those in laboratory.
   (ii) Not sure about what I would have done.
   (iii) Would have sold those to public.

APPENDIX V

Suicidal Tendencies Inventory

Developed by Samuel E. Krug (1989) and locally adapted by Anjana Bhattacharjee and Dr. Sibnath Deb (2002)

Instruction: Eighteen statements are given here. Please read these statements attentively one after another. Three possible responses are given with each statement. For each statement put a correct (√) mark to the response which is appropriate for you.

There is no right or wrong answer in this inventory. Please respond to all the items without any hesitation. Don't spend much time on any one of the statements, but give the answer, which seems to describe you best. Your responses will be kept confidential. If' you feel any difficulty please tell me.

Name:...

Age:... Sex:...

Education:............................... Occupation:............................

Address:...

....

1. **Sometimes I feel that my nerves are breaking into pieces.**
   (i) Yes, I think so.
   (ii) I am not sure.
   (iii) No, I don't think so.
2. **I don't feel physically fit therefore I cannot do my daily work properly.**
   (i) Yes, most of the time I cannot
   (ii) Sometimes I cannot
   (iii) No, in my case it happens very rarely.
3. **I am waiting for the interesting things of life which I can enjoy.**
   (i) Yes I am waiting.
   (ii) Uncertain
   (iii) No, I am not waiting.
4. **I don't get excited by seeing any brave person doing any adventurous work.**
   (i) Yes, I don't get excited.
   (ii) Sometimes I feel excited.
   (iii) No, I always feel excited.
5. **I like adventurous work.**
   (i) Yes, I like very much.
   (ii) I don't like too much.
   (iii) I don't like at all.
6. **I feel disguised to think to go to hospital even when I am sick.**
   (i) Yes, I feel disguised.
   (ii) I don't feel disguised too much
   (iii) I don't feel disguised at all.
7. **Rarely I feel sad and depressed.**
   (i) Yes rarely I feel so.
   (ii) Sometimes I feel so.
   (iii) No, often I feel sad and depressed.
8. **After waking up in the morning I don't get sufficient energy to start the day properly.**
   (i) Yes, I don't get sufficient energy to start the day.
   (ii) I am not sure about this.
   (iii) No, I get sufficient energy.

9. I scare of the thought that no one loves me truly.
(i) Yes, often I scare.
(ii) Rarely I scare
(iii) No, I don't scare at all.

10. I feel frustrated and unnecessary to talk to others.
(i) Yes, I feel so.
(ii) Sometimes I feel so.
(iii) No, I don't feel so.

11. My stomach is very week and I easily get constipation.
(i) Yes, I easily get constipation.
(ii) Sometimes I get constipation.
(iii) No, I don't easily get constipation.

12. I don't think that people misbehave with me.
(i) Yes, I don't think so.
(ii) Uncertain.
(iii) No, I don't think that people misbehave with me.

13. I never think myself so much active that like some people I can stay without sleeping for two/three days at a time.
(i) Yes, I never think myself that much active.
(ii) Uncertain
(iii) No, I think myself that much active.

14. Criticism easily hurts me and makes me depressed.
(i) Yes, often it happens with me.
(ii) Sometimes it happens with me.
(iii) No, never it happens with me.

15. I don't mind if anyone does not respond to me while talking to them.
(i) Yes, most of the time I don't mind.
(ii) Sometimes I don't mind.
(iii) No, always I mind if anyone doesn't respond to me.

16. I don't believe that certain things (seeing a black cat) can bring bad luck in my life.
(i) Yes, I don't believe at all.
(ii) Uncertain.
(iii) No, I always believe that the sight of certain things can bring bad luck in my life.

17. **When I am in a holly place or some other place where I have to maintain silence, I feel afraid that I may break the silence by shouting.**
    (i) Often I feel so.
    (ii) Sometimes I feel so.
    (iii) No, I never think so.
18. **I can feel the better side of life and also can enjoy my work.**
    (i) Yes, I can.
    (ii) Sometimes I can.
    (iii) No, I can't.

Bibliography

Abi Daoud, M.S., Dooley J.M., and Gordon K.E. (2004). Depression in Parents of Children with Duchenne Muscular Dystrophy. *Pediatr Neurol*; 31(1):16-9.

Akiskal, H. S., Maser, J. D., Zeller, P. J., Endicott, J., Coryell, W., Keller, M. B., Warshaw, M., Clayton, P.J., and Goodwin, F. K. (1995). Switching from "Unipular" to Bipolar II: An 11 Years Prospective Study of Clinical and Temperamental Predictors in 559 patients. *Archives of General Psychiatry*; 52, 114-123.

Alexander, B., Brewin, C.R., Vearnals, S., Wolff, G., and Leff, J. (1999). An Investigation of Shame and Guilt in a Depressed Sample. *Br J Med Psychol*; 72 (Pt 3): 323-38.

Allgood-Merten, B., Lewinsohn, P.M., and Hops, H. (1990). Sex Differences and Adolescent Depression. *Journal of Abnormal Psychiatry*; 99, 55-63.

Alvidrez, J., and Azocar F. (1999). Self-Recognition of Depression in Public Care Women's Clinic Patients. *J Womens Health Gend Based Med.*; 8(8): 1063-71.

Andrews, B., and Brown, G.W. (1988). Social Support, Onset of Depression and Personality: An Exploratory Analysis. *Social Psychiatry and Psychiatric Epidemiology*; 23-99-108.

Andrews, B., and Brown, G.W., and Creasey, L. (1990). Intergenerational Links between Psychiatric Disorder between Mothers and Daughters: The Role of Parenting Experiences. *Journal of Child Psychology and Psychiatry*; 31, 1115-1129.

Angold, A., and Costello, E. J. (1993). Depressive Co-morbidity in Children and Adolescents: Empirical, Theoretical, and Methodological Issues. *American Journal of Psychiatry*; 150, 1779-1791.

Bailey et al., (1996). Mediators of Depression in adults with Diabetes. *Clin Nurs Res*; 5(1): 28-42.

Barnett, P.A., and Gotlib, I.H. (1988). Psychological Functioning and Depression: Distinguishing among Antecedents, Concomitants, and Consequences. *Psychological Bulletin*; 104, 97-126.

Beck, A.T. (1967). *Depression: Clinical, Experimental, and Theoretical Aspects;* New York: Harper and Row.

Beekman, A.T., Deeg, D.J., Smit, J.H., Comijs, H.C., Braam, A.W., De Beurs, E, and Van Tilburg, W. (2004). Dysthymia In Later Life: A Study in the Community. *J Affect Disord;* 2004; 81(3):191-9.

Bienvenu, O.J., Samuels, J.F., Costa, P.T., Reti, I.M., Eaton, W.W., and Nestadt, G. (2004). Anxiety and Depressive Disorders and The Five-Factor Model of Personality: A Higher and Lower Order Personality Trait Investigation in a Community Sample. *Depress Anxiety;* 20(2): 92-97.

Bifulco, A.T., Brown, G.W., and Adler, Z. (1991). Early Sexual Abuse and Clinical Depression in Adult Life. *British Journal of Psychiatry;* 159, 115-122.

Bifulco, A.T., Brown, G.W., and Harries, T.O. (1987). Childhood Loss of Parents, Lack of Adequate Parental Care and Adult Depression: A Replication. *Journal of Affective Disorders;* 12, 115-128.

Bisschop, M.I., Kriegsman, D.M., Beekman, A.T., and Deeg, D.J. (2004). Chronic Diseases and Depression: The Modifying Role of Psychosocial Resources. *Soc. Sci. Med.;* 59(4): 721-33.

Blatt, et al., (1991). A Cognitive Morphology of Psychopathology. *J. Nerv. Ment. Dis.;* 179, 449-458.

Blatt, S. J., and Hommen, E. (1992). Parent Child Interaction in The Etiology of Dependent and Self Critical Depression. *Clinical Psychology Review;* 12, 47-91.

Blazer, D.G., Kessler, R.C., Mcgonagle, K.A., and Swartz, M.S. (1994). The Prevalence and Distribution of Major Depression in a National Community Sample: The National Comorbidity Survey. *American Journal of Psychiatry;* 151, 979-986.

Bodlund, O. (2000). Most Depressed Patients Can Be Treated in Primary Health Care. *Lakartidningen;* 97(11): 1244-9.

Bookless, C, Mcfarlane, A, and Clayer, J. (2002). Personal Appraisal of The Experience of a Depressive Disorder. *Br J Med Psychol;* 74 Part 3:399-412.

Bornstein, R.F. (1992). The Dependent Personality: Developmental, Social, and Clinical Perspectives. Psychological Bulletin; 112, 3-23.

Bowlby, J. (1981). *Attachment and Loss: Vol.3. Loss: Sadness and Depression;* Harmondsworth, UK: Penguin.

Bowlby, J. (1978). *Attachment and Loss: Vol.2. Separation: Anxiety and Anger*. Harmondsworth, UK: Penguin.

Bromberger, J.T. (2004). A Psychosocial Understanding of Depression in Women: For the Primary Care Physician. *J Am Med Womens Assoc; 59*(3): 198-206.

Brook, J.S., Schuster, E., Zhangc. (2004). Cigarette Smoking and Depressive Symptoms: A Longitudinal Study of Adolescents and Young Adults. *Psychol Rep*: 95(1): 159-166.

Brown, G.R., and Anderson, B. (1991). Psychiatric Morbidity in Adult Inpatients with Childhood Histories of Sexual and Physical Abuse. *American Journal of Psychiatry;* 148, 55-61.

Brown, G.W., and Harries, T.O. (1993). Aetiology of Anxiety and Depressive Disorders in an Inner-City Population: 1. Early Adversity. *Psychological Medicine*; 23, 143-154.

Brown, G.W., and Harris, T.O. (1978). *Social Origins of Depression: A Study of Psychiatric Disorders in Women;* New York: Free Press.

Brummett, B.H., Barefoot, J.C., Siegler, I.C., and Steffens.D.C. (2000). Relation of Subjective and Received Social Support to Clinical and Self-Report Assessments of Depressive Symptoms in an Elderly Population. *J Affect Disord*; 61 (1-2):41-50.

Buckwald, A.M. and Rudick-Davis, D. (1993). The Symptoms of Major Depression. *Journal of Abnormal Psychology*; 102, 197-205.

Burke, K.C., Burke, J.D., Rae, D., and Regier, D.A. (1991). Comparing Age at Onset of Major Depression and Other Psychiatric Disorders by Birth Cohorts in Five US Community Populations. *Archives of General Psychiatry*; 48, 789-795.

Burke, K.C., Burke, J.D., Regier, D.A., and Rae, D.S. (1990). Age at Onset of Selected Mental Disorders in Five Community Populations. *Archives of General Psychiatry*; 47, 511-518.

Burnam, M. A., Stein, J.A., Golding, J.M., Seigal, J.M., Sorenson, S. B., Forsythe, A.B., and Telles, C.A. (1988). Sexual Assault and Mental Disorders in a Community Population. *Journal of Consulting and Clinical Psychology*; 56, 843-850.

Carlson, G.A., and Cantwell, D.P. (1980). Unmasking Masked Depression in Children and Adolescent. *American Journal of Psychiatry*; 137, 445-449.

Carlson, G.A., and Kashani, J.H. (1988). Phenomenology of Major Depression from Childhood through Adulthood: Analysis of Three Studies. *American Journal of Psychiatry*; 145, 1222-1225.

Casper, R.C. (1998) Depression and Eating Disorders. *Depress Anxiety*; 8 Suppl 1:96-104.

Cattell, R.B., Eber, H.W., and Tatsuoka, M.M. (1970). *Hand Book For the Sixteen Personality Factor Questionnaire (16 PF)*. Champaign; III. : IPAT.

Clark, D.C. (1995). Epidemiology, Assessment, and Management of Suicide in Depressed Patients. In E.E. Beckham and W.R. Leber (Eds.), *Handbook of Depression (2nd ed.)*; (pp. 526-38). New York: Guilford.

Cloitre, M., Katz, M.M., and Van Praag, H.M. (1993). Psychomotor Agitation and Retardation. Un C.G. Costello (Ed.,), *Synptoms of Depression* (pp.207-226). New York: Wiley.

Coffey, C.E., Wildinson, W.E., Weiner, R.D., Parashos, I. A., Djang, W.T., Webb, M.C., Figiel, G.S., and Spritzer, C.E. (1993). Quantitative Cereblar Anatomy in Depression: A Controlled Magnetic Resonance Imaging Study. *Archives of General Psychiatry; 50, 7-16.*

Cole, D.A., and Mcpherson, A.E. (1993). Relation of Family Subtypes to Adolescent Depression: Implementing a New Family Assessment Strategy. *Journal of Family Psychology*; 7, 119-133.

Cornelius, J.R., Salloum, I.M., Mezzich, J., Cornelius, M.D., Fabrega , H. J, Ehler, J.G., Ulrich, R.F., Thase, M.E., and

Mann, J.J. (1995). Disproportionate Suicidality in Patients with Comorbid Major Depression and Alcoholism. *American Journal of Psychiatry;* 152(3): 358-64.

Coryell, W., Endicott, J., and Keller, M.B. (1991). Predictors of Relapse into Major Depressive Disorder in a Non-Clinical Population. *American Journal of Psychiatry;* 148,1353-1358.

Coryell, W., Endicott, j., Maser, J.D., Keller, M.B., Leon, A.C., and Akishkal, H.S. (1995). Long Term Stability of Polarity Distinctions in the Affective Disorders. *American Journal of Psychiatry;* 152, 385-390.

Coryell, W.,Winokur, G., Shea, T., Maser, J.D., Endicott, J., and Akishkal, H.S. (1994). The Long Term Stability of Depressive Subtypes. *American Journal of Psychiatry;* 151, 199-204.

Costello, C.G. (1982). Social Factors Associated with Depression:A Retrospective Community Study. *Psychological Medicine;* 12, 329-339.

Cox, B.J., Rector, N.A., Bagby, R.M., Swinson, R.P., Levitt, A. J., and Joffe, R.T. (2000). Is Self-Criticism Unique for Depression? A Comparison With Social Phobia. *J Affect Disord;* 57(1-3): 223-8.

Daniels, D., and Moos, R.H. (1990). Assessing Life Stressors and Social Resources Among Adolescents: Applications to Depressed Youth. *Journal of Adolescent Research;* 5, 268-289.

Davies, P.T., and Windle, M. (1997). Gender-Specific Pathways between Maternal Depressive Symptoms, Family Discord, and Adolescent Adjustment. *Delop. Psychol ;* 33(4), 657-68.

DeBonis, M., DeBoeck, P., Lida-Pulik H, Hourtane, M., and Feline, A. (1998). Self-Concept and Mood: A Comparative Study between Depressed Patients with and without Borderline Personality Disorder. *J Affect Disord. ;* 48(2-3): 191-7.

Eiber, R., Puel, M., and Schmitt, L. (1999). Heroin Abuse, Autobiographical Memory and Depression. *Encephale.;* 25(6): 549-57.

Ellen McGrath (2002). Love Needs, Published by Psychology Today: December 1, 2002.

Fadden, G., Bebbington, P.E., and Kuipers, L. (1987). Caring and its Burdens: A Study of the Spouses of Depressed Patients. *British Journal of Psychiatry*; 151, 660-667.

Faedda, G.L., Tondo, L., Teicher, M.H., Baldessarini, R.J., Gelbard, H.A., and Floris, G. F. (1993). Seasonal Mood Disorders: Patterns of Seasonal Recurrence In Mania and Depression. *Archives of General Psychiatry*; 50, 17-23.

Fava, M., Abraham, M., Clancy-Colecchi, K., Pava, J.A., Matthews, J, and Rosenbaum, J.F. (1997). Eating Disorder Symptomatology in Major Depression. *J Nerv Ment Dis*; 185(3): 140-4.

Feighner, J.P., Robins, E., et al., (1972). Diagnostic Criteria for use in Psychiatric Research. *Arch. Gen.Psychiatry*; 26, 56-73.

Flemming, J.E., and Offord, D.R. (1990). Epidemiology of Childhood Depressive Disorders: a Critical Review. *Journal of The American Academy of Child and Adolescent Psychiatry*; 29, 571-580.

Ford, D.E., and Kamerow, D.B. (1989). Epidemiologic Study of Sleep Disturbances and Psychiatric Disorders: An Opportunity for Prevention? *Journal of The American Medical Association*; 262, 1479-1484.

Friedman, A.S., Terras, A., Zhu W., and McCallum, J. (2004). Depression, Negative Self-Image, and Suicidal Attempts as Effects of Substance use and Substance Dependence. *J Addict Dis*; 23(4): 55-71.

Garrison, C.Z., Jackson, K.L., Marstellar, F., Mckeown, R.E., and Addy, C. (1990). A Longitudinal Study of Depressive Symptomatology in Young Adolescents. *Journal of the American Academy of Child and Adolescent Psychiatry*; 29, 581-585.

Gerlsma, C., Emmelkamp, P.M.G., and Arrindell, W.A. (19090). Anxiety, Depression, and Perception of Early Parenting: A Meta-Analysis. *Clinical Psychology Review*; 10, 251-277.

Gershon, E.S. (1990). Genetics. In F.K. Goodwin and K.R.Jamison (Eds.), *Manic Depressive Illness*; New York: Oxford University Press.

Giles, D.E., Jarret, R., Rush, A.J., Biggs, M., and Roffwarg, H.P. (1993). Prospective Assessment of Electroencelographic Sleep in Remitted Major Depressives. Psychiatry Research; 46, 269-284.

Giles, D.E., Roffwarg, H.P., Dahl, R.E., and Kupfer, D.J.(1992). EEG Sleep Abnormalities in Depressed Children: A Hypothesis. Psychiatry Research; 41, 53-63.

Gitlin, M.J. (1996). *The Psychotherapist's Guide to Psychopharcology* (2nd Ed.); New York: Free Press.

Gongora,V.C., Van Der Staak C.P., and Derksen J.J. (2004). Personality Disorders, Depression, and Coping Styles in Argentinean Bulimic Patients. *J Personal Disord*; 18(3): 272-85.

Goodyer, I., and Cooper, P.J. (1993). A Community Study of Depression in Adolescent Girls: II. The Clinical Features of Identified Disorder. *British Journal of Psychiatry*; 163, 374-380.

Gotlib, I.H., and Hammen, C.L. (1992). *Psychological Aspects of Depression: Toward a Cognitive—Interpersonal Integration*; Chichester, UK: Wiley.

Gotlib, I.H., and Lee, C.M. (1990). Children of Depressed Mother: A Review and Directions for Future Research. In C.D. Mccann & N.S. Endler (Eds.), *Depression: New Directions in Theory, Research, and Practice* (pp.187-208). Toronto: Wall & Thompson.

Gotlib, I.H., Mount, J.H., Cordy, N.I., and Whiffen, V.E. (1988). Depression and Perception of Early Parenting: A Longitudinal Investigation. *British Journal of Psychiatry*; 152, 24-27.

Gotlib, I.H., and Whiffen, V.E. (1989). Depression and Marital Functioning: An Examination of Specificity and Gender Differences. *Journal of Abnormal Psychology*; 98, 23-30.

Gotlib, I., Whiffen, V.E., Wallace , P., and Mount, J.H. (1991). A Prospective Investigation of Postpartum Depression: Factors involved in Onset and Recovery. *Journal of Abnormal Psychology*; 100, 122-132.

Greenberg, J. (1982). Suicide Linked to Brain Chemical Deficit. *Science News*; 121, 355.

Gunderson, J.G., Morey, L.C., Stout, R.L., Skodol, A.E., Shea, M.T., Mcglashan, T.H., Zanarini, M.C., Grilo, C.M., Sanislow, C.A., Yen, S., Daversa, M.T., and Bender, D.S. (2004). Major Depressive Disorder and Borderline Personality Disorder Revisited: Longitudinal Interactions. *J Clin Psychiatry*; 65 (8): 1049-56.

Hakkarainen, R., Partonen, T., Haukka, J., Virtamo, J., Albanes,D., and Lonnqvist, J. (2003). Association of Dietary Amino Acids with Low Mood. *Depress Anxiety*; 18(2): 89-94.

Hallfors, D.D., Waller, M.W., Ford, C.A., Halpern, C.T., Brodish, P.H., and Iritani, B.(2004). Adolescent Depression and Suicide Risk Association with Sex and Drug Behaviour. *Am J Prev Med*; 27(3): 224-31.

Hammen, C., Brennan, P.A., and Shih, J.H. (2004). Family Discord and Stress Predictors of Depression and Other Disorders in Adolescent Children of Depressed and Nondepressed Women. *J Am Acad Child Adolesc Psychiatry*; 43(8): 994-1002.

Hammen, C.L. (1991a). Depression Runs in Families: The Social Context of Risk and Resilience in Children of Depressed Mothers. New York: Springer-Verlag.

Hammen, C.L., Burge, D., Daley, S.E., Davila, J., Paley,B., and Rudolph, K.D. (1995). Interpersonal Attachment Cognition and Prediction of Symptomatic Responses to Interpersonal Stress. *Journal of Abnormal Psychology* ; 104, 436-443.

Hammen, C.L., and Rudolph, K.D. (1996). Childhood Depression. In E.J. Mash and R.A.Barkley (Eds.), *Child Psychopathology* (pp. 153-195). New York. Guilford.

Harris, T., Brown, G.W., and Bifulco, A.T. (1986). Loss of Parent in Childhood and Adult Psychiatric Disorder: The Role of Lack of Adequate Parental Care. *Psychological Medicine;* 16, 641-659.

Hayward, P., Wong, G., Bright, J.A., and Lam, D. (2002). Stigma and Self-Esteem in Manic Depression: An Exploratory Study. *J Affect Disord;* 69(1-3): 61-7.

Henriques, J.B., and Devidson, R.J. (1990). Regional Brain Electrical Asymmetries Discriminate between previously

Depressed and Healthy Control Subjects. *Journal of Abnormal Psychology*; 99, 22-31.

Henriques, J.B., and Devidson, R.J. (1991). Left Frontal Hypoactivation in Depression. *Journal of Abnormal Psychology; 100*, 535-545.

Hirschfeld, R.M.A., Klerman, G.L., Andreasen, N.C., Clayton, P.J., and Keller, M.B. (1986). Psycho-social Predictors of Chronicity in Depressed Patients. British Journal of Psychiatry; 148, 648-654.

Hirschfeld, R.M.A., Klerman, G.L., Clayton, P.J., and Keller, M.B. (1983). Personality and Depression: Empirical Findings. *Archives of General Psychiatry* ; 40, 993-998.

Hollon, S.D. DeRubies, R. J., and Evans, M. D. (1996). Cognitive Therapy in the Treatment and Prevention of Depression. In P.M. Salkovskis (Ed.), *Frontiers of Cognitive Therapy*. (pp. 293-317). New York: Guilford.

Hong, J. P., Samuels, J., Bienvenu, O.J., .3rd, Cannistraro, P., Grados, M., Riddle, M.A., Liang, K.Y., Cullen, B., Hoehn-Saric, R., and Nestadt, G. (2004). Clinical Correlates of Recurrent Major Depression In obsessive-Compulsive Disorder. *Depress Anxiety*; 20(2): 86-91.

Howes, M.J., Hokanson, J.E., and Loewenstein, D.A. (1985). Induction of Depressive Affect After Prolonged Exposure to a Mildly Depressed Individual. *J. Pers. Soc. Psycho.*; 49, 1110-13.

Intili, H., and Nier D. (1998). Self-Esteem and Depression in Men Who Present With Erectile Dysfunction. *Urol Nurs.* ; 18(3): 185-7, 208.

Iqbal, Z., Birchwood, M., Chadwick, P., and Trower, P. (2000). Cognitive Approach to Depression and Suicidal Thinking in Psychosis. Testing the Validity of a Social Ranking Model. *Br J Psychiatry*; 177:522-8.

Jacobsen, F.M., Wher, T.A., Sack, D.A., James, S.P., and Rosenthal, N. E. (1986). Seasonal Affective Disorder: A Review of the Syndrome and Its Public Health Implications. *American Journal of Public Health*; 77, 57-60.

Jambunathan, Jaylakshmi (1992). Socio-Cultural Factors. In Depression in Asian Indian Women, *Psychological Abstract*; Vol. 80; 4485.

Jawor, M., Dimter, A., Marek, K., Dudek, D., Wojtys, A., Szproch, A. (2001). Anxiety-Depressive Disorder in Women after Hysterectomy. Own Study. *Psychiatr Pol*; 35(5): 771-80.

Joiner, T. E., and Metalsky, G.I. (1995). A Prospective test of an Integrative Interpersonal Theory of Depression. A Naturalistic Study of College Roommates. *J. Pers. Soc . Psycho; 69*(4), 778-88.

Joyce, P.R., and Paykel, E.S. (1989). Predictors of Drug Response in Depression. *Achieves of General Psychiatry* ; 46, 89-99.

Karson, S., and O, Dell, J.W. (1976). *A Guide to the Chemical Use of the 16 PF*. Chaimpaign; III. : P IPAT.

Kashani, J.H., and Carlson, G. A. (1987). Seriously Depressed Preschoolers. *American Journal of Psychiatry*; 144, 348-350.

Kashani, J.H., Holcomb, W.R., and Orvaschel, H. (1986). Depression and Depressive Symptoms in Preschool Children from the General Population. *American Journal of Psychiatry*; 143, 1138-1143.

Kashani, J.H., Rosenberg, T.K. and Reid, J.C. (1989). Developmental Perspectives in Child and Adolescents Depressive Symptoms. In a Community Sample. *American Journal of Psychiatry*; 146, 871-875.

Kaslow, N.J., Deering, C.G., and Racusin, G.R. (1994). Depressed Children and their Families. *Clinical Psychology Review;* 14,39-59.

Kendler, K.S., Neale, M.C., Kessler, R.C., Health, A.C., and Eaves, L.J. (1992). A Population based Twin Study of Major Depression in Women. *Achieves of General Psychiatry*; 49, 257-266.

Kendler, K.S., Neale, M.C., Kessler, R.C., Health, A.C., and Eaves, L.J. (1993). A Longitudinal Twin Study of 1-Year Prevalence of Major Depression in Women. *Achieves of General Psychiatry*; 50, 843-852.

Kessler, R.C., and Magee, W.J. (1993). Childhood Adversities and Adult Depression: Basic Patterns of Association in a US National Survey. *Psychological Medicine*; 23, 679-690.

Kessler, R.C., Mc.Gonagle, K.A., Zhao, S., Nelson, C.B., Hughes, M., Eshleman, S., Wittchen, H.U., and Kendler, K.S. (1994).

Lifetime and 12-Month Prevalence of DSM-III-R Psychiatric Disorders in the United States: Results From the National Comorbidity Survey. *Arch. Gen. Psychiat.* ; 51,8-19.

King, C.A., Katz, S.H., Ghaziuddin, N., Brand, E., Hill, E., and Mcgovern, L. (1997). Diagnosis and Assessment of Depression and Suicidality using the NIMH Diagnostic Interview Schedule for Children (DISC-2.3). *J Abnorm Child Psychol*; 25(3): 173-81.

Klein, D.N., Riso, L.P., Donaldson, S.K., Schwartz, J.E., Anderson, R.L., Ouimette, P.C., Lizardi, H., and Aronson, T.A. (1995). Family Study of Early-Onset Dysthymia. *Achieves of General Psychiatry*; 52, 487-496.

Klein, D.N., Taylor, E.B., Dickstein, S., and Harding, K. (1988). Primary Early-Onset Dysthymia: Comparison with Primary Nonbipolar Nonchronic Major Depression On Demographic, Clinical, Familial, Personality, and Socio Environmental Characteristics and Short-Term Outcome. *Journal of Abnormal Psychology; 97, 387-398.*

Klerman, G.L., and Weissman, M.M. (1989). Increasing Rates of Depression. *Journal of the American Medical Association;* 261, 2229-2235.

Klinger, E. (1993). Loss of Interest. In C.G. Costello (Ed.), *Symptoms of Depression* (pp.43-62). New York: Wiley.

Kobak, R.R., Sudler, N., and Gamble, W. (1991). Attachment and Depressive Symptoms during Adolescence: A Developmental Pathways Analysis. *Development and Psychopathology*; 3, 461-474.

Kovacs, M., Akiskal, M., Akiskal, H.S., Gatsonis, C., and Parrone, P.L. (1994). Childhood-Onset Dysthymic Disorder: Clinical Features and Prospective Naturalistic Outcome. *Archives of General Psychiatry*; 51, 365-374.

Kuo, W.H., Gallo, J.J., and Eaton, W.W. (2004). Hopelessness, Depression, Substance Disorder, and Suicidality-A 13-Year Community-Based Study. *Soc. Psychiatr. Epidemiol; 39*(6): 497-501.

Kupfer, D.J., and Thase, N.E. (1983). the use of The Sleep Laboratory in the Diagnosis of Affective Disorders. *Psychiatric Clinic of North America*; 5, 3-25.

Lam, D., Schuck, N., Smith, N., Farmer, A., and Checkley, S. (2003). Response Style, Interpersonal Difficulties and Social Functioning in Major Depressive Disorder. *J Affect Disord;* 75(3): 279-83.

Lauer, C., Schreiber, W., Holsboer, F., and Krieg, J.C. (1995). In Quest of Identifying Vulnerability Markers for Psychiatric Disorders by All-Night Polysomnography. *Achieves of General Psychiatry; 52, 145-153.*

Lee, D.T., Chan S.S., Sahota, D.S., Yip, A.S., Tsui, M., and Chung, T.K. (2004). A Prevalence Study of Antenatal Depression among Chinese Women. *J Affect Disord*; 82(1): 93-9.

Lewinsohn, P.M., Hops, H., Roberts, R.E., Seeley, J.R., and Andrews, J.A. (1993). Adolescent Psychopathology: I. Prevalence and Incidence of Depression and Other DSM-III-R Disorders in High School Students, *Journal of Abnormal Psychology*; 102,133-144.

Lichtenberger, C.M., Martin Ginis, K.A., Mackenzie, C.L., and Mccartney, N. (2003). Body Image and Depressive Symptoms as Correlates of Self-Reported Versus Clinician-Reported Physiologic Function. *J Cardiopulm Rehabil;* 23(1):53-9.

Lizerdi, H., Klein, D.N., Ouimette, P.C., Riso, L.P., Anderson, R.L., and Donaldson, S.K. (1995). Reports of the Childhood Home Environment in Early-Onset Dysthymia and Episodic Major Depression. *Journal of Abnormal Psychology;* 104, 132-139.

Lobentanz, I.,S., Asenbaum, S., Vass, K., Sauter, C., Klosch, G., Kollegger, H., Kristoferitsch, W., and Zeitlhofer, J. (2004). Factors Influencing Quality of Life in Multiple Sclerosis Patients: Disability, Depressive Mood, Fatigue and Sleep Quality. *Acta Neurol Scand;* 110(1): 6-13.

Lynch, T.R., Mendelson T., Robins, C.J., Krishnan, K.R., George, L.K., Johnson, C.S., and Blazer, D.G. (1999). Perceived Social Support among Depressed Elderly, Middle-Aged, and Young-Adult Samples: Cross-Sectional and Longitudinal Analyses. *J Affect Disord*; 55(2-3): 159-70.

Manwell, L.B., Czabala, J.C., Ignaczak, M., and Mundt, M.P. (2004). Correlates of Depression among Heavy Drinkers in Polish Primary Care Clinics. *Int J Psychiatry Med.*; 34(2): 165-78

Margc, Geofferey, M., Greenberg, Roger, P., Fisher, Seymeur and Dewan, Mantosh (1993). A Direct Comparison of the Defence Mechanisms of Non-Depressed People and Psychiatric in Patients. *Psychological Abstract*; Vol. 80; 4485.

Maris.R. W., Berman, A.L., Maltsberger, J.T. and Yufit, R.I. (1992). *Assessment and Prediction of Suicide.* New York: Guilford.

Marmorstein, N.R., Malone, S.M., and Iacono, W.G. (2004). Psychiatric Disorders among Offspring of Depressed Mothers: Associations with Paternal Psychopathology. *Am J Psychiatry*; 161(9): 1588-94.

Martin, G., Bergen, H.A., Roeger, L., and Allison, S. (2004). Depression in Young Adolescents: Investigations Using 2 and 3 Factor Versions of the Parental Bonding Instrument. *J Nerv Ment Dis*; 192(10): 650-657.

McGuffin, P., Ketz, R., Watkins, S., and Rutherford, J. (1996). A Hospital-Based Twin Register of the Habitability of DSM-IV Unipolar Depression. *Achieves of General Psychiatry*; 53, 129-136.

McNeal, E.T., and Cimbolic, P. (1986). Anti-depressent and Biochemical Theories of Depression. *Psychological Bulletin*; 99, 361-374.

Menzies, V. (2000). Depression in Schizophrenia: Nursing Care as a Generalized Resistance Resource. *Issues Ment Health Nurs.* ; 21(6): 605-17.

Mitchell, J.R., Mccauley, E., Burke, P.M. and Moss, S.J. (1988). Phenomenology of Depression in Children and Adolescents. *Child and Adolescent Psychiatry*; 27, 2-20.

Murry, L., Fiori-Cowley, A., Hooper, R., and Cooper, P. (1996). The Impact of Postnatal Depression and Associated Adversity on Early Mother-Infant Interactions and Later infant Outcomes. *Child Develop.* ; 67(5), 2512-26.

Neiderehe, G. and Schneider. (1998). Treatments for Depression and Anxiety in the Aged. In P.E. Nathan and J.M.Gorman, *A Guide to Treatments that Work.* (pp. 270-87). New York: Oxford University Press.

Nelson, G. (1982). Parental Death During Childhood and Adult Depression: Some Additional Data. *Social Psychiatry*; 17, 37-42.

Nurnberger, J., and Gershon, E.S. (1984). Genetics of Affective Disorders. In R. Post and J. Ballenger (Eds.), *Neurobiology of Mood Disorder* (pp.76-101). Baltimore: Williams and Wilkins.

O'Connor, D.W., Rosewarne, R, and Bruce, A. (2001). Depression In Primary Care. 1: Elderly Patients' Disclosure of Depressive Symptoms to their Doctors. *Int Psychogeriatr*; 13(3): 359-65.

O'Hara, M.W., Schlechte, J.A., Lewis, D.A., and Varner, M.W. (1991). Controlled Prospective Study of Postpartum Mood Disorders: Psychological, Environmental, and Hormonal Variables. *Journal of Abnormal Psychology*; 100, 63-73.

O'Hara, M.W., Zekoski, E.M., Philipps, L.H., and Wright, E. J. (1990). Controlled Prospective Study of Postpartum Mood Disorders: Comparison of Child Bearing and Non-Child Bearing Women; *Journal of Abnormal Psychology*; 99, 3-15.

Ohayon, M.M. (2004). Specific Characteristics of The Pain/ Depression Association in the General Population. *J Clin Psychiatry*; 65 Suppl 12:5-9.

Olley, B.O., Seedat, S., Nei, D.G., and Stein, D.J. (2004). Predictors of Major Depression in Recently Diagnosed Patients With HIV/AIDS In South Africa. *AIDS Patient Care STDS*; 18(8): 481-7.

Oquendo, M.A., Friedman, J.H., Grunebaum, M.F., Burke, A., Silver, J.M., and Mann, J.J. (2004). Suicidal Behaviour and Mild Traumatic Brain Injury In Major Depression. *J Nerv Ment Dis*; 192(6): 430-4.

Oral, E.T., and Vahip, S. (2004). Bipolar Depression: An Overview. : *I Drugs; 7*(9): 846-50.

Oren, D.A., and Rosenthal, N.E. (1992). Seasonal Affective Disorders. In E.S. Paykel (Ed.), *Handbook of Affective Disorders* (2nd Ed.), (pp. 551-67). New York: Guilford.

O'Sullivan C. (2004). The Psychosocial Determinants of Depression: A Lifespan Perspective. *J Nerv Ment Dis.*; 192(9): 585-94.

Otsuki, T.A. (2003). Substance Use, Self-Esteem and Depression among Asian American Adolescents. *J Drug Educ.*; 33(4): 369-90.

Pasquini, M., Picardi, A., Biondi, M., Gaetano, P., and Morosini, P. (2004). Relevance of Anger and Irritability in Outpatients with Major Depressive Disorder. *Psychopathology;* 37(4): 155-60.

Petersen, A.C., Sarigiani, P.A., and Kennedy, R.E. (1991). Adolescent Depression: Why More Girls? *Journal of Youth and Adolescence*; 20, 247-271.

Philipps, L.H.C., and O' Hara, M.W. (1991). Prospective Study of Postpartum Depression: 4 and ½ Year Follow-Up of Women and Children. *Journal of Abnormal Psychology*; 100, 151-155.

Phillips J., Carpenter, K., and Nunes, E. (2004). Suicide Risk in Depressed Methadone-Maintained Patients: Associations with Clinical and Demographic Characteristics. *Am J Addict;* 13(4): 327-32.

Pincus, T., Griffith, J., Pearce, S., and Isenberg, D. (1996). Prevalence of Self-Reported Depression in Patients with Rheumatoid Arthritis. *Br J Rheumatol;* 35(9): 879-83.

Plomin, R., DeFries, J.C., McClearn, G. E., and Rutter, M. (1997). *Behaviour Genetics (3rd Ed.)*; New York: W.H.Freeman.

Powell, K .B., and Miklowitz, D.J. (1994). Frontal Lobe Dysfunction in the Affective Disorders. *Clinical Psychology Review;* 14, 525-546.

Power, M.J., Cameron, C.M., and Dalgleish, T. (1996). Emotional Priming in Clinically Depressed Subjects. *J.Affect Disord;* 26; 38, (1): 1-11.

Prochazka, H., and Agren, H. (2003). Self-Rated Aggression and Cerebral Monoaminergic Turnover. Sex Differences In Patients with Persistent Depressive Disorder. *Eur. Arch. Psychiatry Clin. Neurosci*; 253(4): 185-92.

Rada, R.E., and Johnson-Leong, C. (2004). Stress, Burnout, Anxiety and Depression among Dentists. *J Am Dent Assoc*; 135(6): 788-94.

Reiche, E.M., Nunes, S.O., and Morimoto, H.K. (2004). Stress, Depression, The Immune System, and Cancer. *Lancet Oncol*; 5(10): 617-25.

Reynolds, C.F., and Kupfer, D.J. (1987). Sleep Research in Affective Illness: State of The Art Circa 1987. *Sleep*; 10, 199-215.

Rose, D.T., Abramson, L.Y., Hodulik, C.J., Halberstadt, L., and Leff, G. (1994). Heterogeneity of Congenetive Style among Depressed Inpatients. *Journal of Abnormal Psychology*; 103, 419-429.

Rosenfarb, I.S., Becker, J., and Khan, A. (1994). Perceptions of Parental and Peer Attachments with Mood Disorders. *Journal of Abnormal Psychology*; 103, 637-644.

Rosenfarb, I.S., Becker, J., Khan, A., and Mintz, J. (1998). Dependency and Self-Criticism in Bipolar and Unipolar Depressed Women. *Br J Clin Psychol.*; 37 (Pt 4): 409-14.

Rush, A.J., and Weissenburger, J.E. (1994). Melancholic Symptom Features and DSM-IV. *American Journal of Psychiatry*; 151, 489-498.

Ryan, N.D., Puig-Antich, J., Ambrosini, P., Rabinovich, H., Robinson, D., Nelson, B., Iyenger, S., and Twomey, J. (1987). The Clinical Picture of Major Depression in Children and Adolescents. *Archives of General Psychiatry*; 44, 854-861.

Ryan, N.D., Williamson, D.E., Iyengar, S., Orvaschel, H., Reich, T., Dahl, R.E., and Puig-Antich, J. (1992). A Secular Increase in Child and Adolescent Onset Affective Disorder. *Journal of The American Academy of Child and Adolescent Psychiatry*; 31, 600-605.

Sands, J.R., and Harrow, M. (1994). Psychotic Unipolar Depression at Follow-Up: Factors Related to Psychosis in The Affective Disorders. *American Journal of Psychiatry*; 151, 995-1000.

Schildkraut, J.J. (1965). Catecholamine Hypothesis of Affective Disorder: A Review of Supporting Evidence. American *Journal of Psychiatry*; 122, 509-522.

Schrag, A., Jahanshahi, M., and Quinn, N.P. (2001). What Contributes to Depression in Parkinson's Disease? *Psychol Med*; 31(1): 65-73.

Sen, B. (2004). Adolescent Propensity for Depressed Mood and Help Seeking: Race and Gender Differences. *J Ment Health Policy Econ.* ; 7(3): 133-145.

Serretti, A., Cavallini M.C., Macciardi F., Namia,C., Franchini, L., Souery, D., Lipp, O., Bauwens, F., Smeraldi, E., and Mendlewicz, J. (1999). Social Adjustment and Self-Esteem in Remitted Patients With Mood Disorders. *Eur Psychiatry*; 14(3): 137-42.

Shelton, R.C., Hollon, S.D., Purdon, S.E., and Loosen, P.T. (1991). Bilogical and Psychological Aspects of Depression. *Behaviour Therapy*; 22, 201-228.

Sheppard, L.C., and Teasdale, J.D.(1996). Depressive Thinking: Changes in Schematic Mental Models of Self and World. *Psychol Med*; 26(5):1043-51.

Sherbourne, C.D., Hays, R.D., and Wells, K.B. (1995). Personal and Psychosocial Risk Factors For Physical and Mental Health Outcomes and Course of Depression among Depressed Patients. *Journal of Consulting and Clinical Psychology*; 63, 345-355.

Sher, L., Oquendo, M. A., Galfalvy, H.C., Cooper T.B., and Mann J.J. (2004). Age Effects On Cortisol Levels in Depressed Patients With and without Comorbid Post-Traumatic Stress Disorder, and Healthy Volunteers. *J Affect Disord.*; 82 (1): 53-9.

Shnek, Z.M., Irvine, J., Stewart,D., and Abbey, S. (2001). Psychological Factors and Depressive Symptoms in Ischemic Heart Disease. *Health Psychol.*; 20(2): 141-5.

Sieber, L.J., and Devis, K.L. (1985). Overview: Toward A Dysregulation Hypothesis of Depression. *American Journal of Psychiatry*; 142, 1017-1031.

Silverman, M. M. (1997). Current Controversies in Suicidology . in R.W. Maris, M. M. Silverman, and S. S. Canetton (Eds.), *Review of Suicidology*, 1997. (pp. 1-21). New York: Guilford.

Silverstone, P.H., Lemay, T., Elliott, J., Hsu, V., and Starko, R.(1996). The Prevalence of Major Depressive Disorder and Low Self-Esteem in Medical Inpatients. *Can J Psychiatry*; 41(2): 67-74.

Skidmore, S. (1977). Translating Psychological Profiles into Treatment Procedure. Ch. 6 in Krug, S.E. (Ed.) *Psychological Assessment in Medicine*; Champaign; Ill. : IPAT.

Smith, A.L., and Weissman, M.M. (1992). Epidemiology. In E.S. Paykel (Ed.,), *Handbook of Affective Disorders* (pp. 111-129). New York: Guilford.

Sorenson, S.B., Rutter, C.M., and Aneshensel, C.S. (1991). Depression in the Community: An Investigation Into Age of Onset. *Journal of Consulting Clinical Psychology*; 59, 541-546.

Spitzer, R.L., Endicott, J., and Robins, E. (1978). Research Diagnostic Criteria for a Selected Group of Functional Disorder. New York: Biometric Research, Institute of Psychistry.

Starkstein, S.E., and Robinson, R.G. (1991). The Role of The Frontal Lobes in affective Disorders Following Stroke. In H.L.Levin, H.M.Eisenberg, and A.L.Benton (Eds.), *Frontal Lobe Function and Dysfunction* (pp. 288-303).New York: Oxford University Press.

Starling, J., Rey, J.M., and Simpson, J.M. (2004). Depressive Symptoms and Suicidal Behaviour: Changes with time in an Adolescent Clinic Cohort. *Aust. N Z J Psychiatry*; 38(9): 732-7.

Stern, M.I., Herron, W.G., Primavera, L.H., and Kakuma T. (1997). Interpersonal Perceptions of Depressed and Borderline Inpatients. *J. Clin Psychol*; 53(1): 41-9.

Sullivan, M., Levy, W.C., Russo J.E., and Spertus, J.A. (2004). Depression and Health Status in Patients with Advanced Heart Failure: A Prospective Study in Tertiary Care. *J Card Fail*; 10(5): 390-6.

Svanborg, P., and Asberg, M. (2001). A Comparison Between The Beck Depression Inventory (BDI) and the Self-Rating Version of The Montgomery Asberg Depression Rating Scale (MADRS). *J Affect Discord*; 64(2-3): 203-16.

Svanborg, P., and Ekselius, L. (2003). Self-Assessment of DSM-IV Criteria for Major Depression in Psychiatric Out-And Inpatients. *Nord J Psychiatry*; 57(4): 291-6.

Thase, M.E., and Howland, R.H. (1995). Biological Processes in Depression: An Updated Review and Integration. In E.E. Beckham and W.R. Leber(Eds.), *Handbook of Depression* (2nd Ed.). (pp. 213-279). New York: Guilford.

Thase, M.E., Reynolds III, C.F., Frank, E., Simons, A.D., McGeary, J., Fasiczka, A.L., Garamoni, G.G., Jennings, R., and Kupfer, D.J. (1994). Do Depressed Men And Women Respond Similarly to Cognitive Behaviour Therapy? American *Journal of Psychiatry*; 151, 500-505.

Tsutsumi, A., Izutsu, T., Akramul Islam, M.D., Amed, J.U., Nakahara, S., Takagi, F., and Wakai, S. (2004). Depressive Status of Leprosy Patients in Bangladesh: Association with Self-Perception of Stigma. *Leprrev*; 75(1): 57-66.

Useda, J.D., Duberstein, P.R., Conner, K.R., and Conwell, Y. (2004). Personality and Attempted Suicide in Depressed Adults 50 Years of Age and Older: A Facet Level Analysis. *Compr. Psychiatry*; 45(5): 353-61.

Wallace, J., and O'Hara, M.W. (1992). Increases in Depressive Symptomatology in the Rural Elderly: Results From a Cross-Sectional and Longitudinal Study. *Journal of Abnormal Psychology*, 101, 398-404.

Watkins, E., and Teasdale, J.D. (2004). Adaptive and Maladaptive Self-Focus in Depression. *J Affect Disord*; 82(1): 1-8.

Watts, F.N. (1993). Problems of Memory and Concentration. In C.G.Costello (Ed.), *Symptoms of Depression* (pp. 113-140). New York: Wiley.

Weiner, R.D., and Coffey, C.E. (1988). Indication for use of Electro-convulsive Therapy. In A. Frances and R. Hales (Eds.), *Review of Psychiatry* (Vol.7, pp. 458-481); Washington, DC: American Psychiatric Press.

Weissman, M.M., Leaf, P., and Bruce, M.L. (1987). Single Parent Women: A Community Study. *Social Psychiatry*; 22, 29-36.

Weissman, M.M., and Olfson, M. (1995). Depression in Women: Implications for Health Care Research. *Science*; 269, 799-801.

Werth J.L. Jr. (2004). The Relationships among Clinical Depression, Suicide, and other Actions that may Hasten Death. *Behav Sci Law*; 22(5): 627.

Whiffen, V.E., and Gotlib, I.H. (1993). Comparison of Postpartum and Non-Postpartum Depression: Clinical Presentation, Psychiatric History, and Psychosocial

Functioning. *Journal of Consulting and Clinical Psychology;* 61, 485-494.

Wilcox, H.C., and Anthony, J.C. (2004). Child and Adolescent Clinical Features as Forerunners of Adult-Onset Major Depressive Disorder: Retrospective Evidence From an Epidemiological Sample. *J Affect Discord.* ; 82(1): 9-20.

Williams, J.B., Spitzer, R.L., Linzer, M., Kroenke, K., Hahn, S.R., Degruy, F.V., and Lazev, A. (1995). Gender Differences in Depression in Primary Care. *Am J Obstet Gynecol;* 173(2): 654-9.

Wing, J.K., Cooper, J.E., et al.,(1974). *Measurements and Classification of Psychiatric Symptoms: An Instrumental Manual for PSE and CATEGO Programe.* New York: Cambridge University Press.

Wilson, M.R., Coleman, A.L., Yu F., Fong Sasaki, I., Bing, E.G., and Kim, M.H. (2002). Depression in Patients with Glaucoma as Measured by Self-Report Surveys; 109(5): 1018-22.

Winokour, G. (1979). Unipolar Depression: It is Divisible into Autonomous Sub-Types. *Arch Gen Psychiatry;* 36, 47-52.

Winokur, G., Coryell, W., Keller, M.B., Endicott, J., and Leon, A.C. (1995). A Family Study of Manic-Depressive (Bipolar I) Disease: Is it a Distinct Illness Separable from Primary Unipolar Depression? *Archives of General Psychiatry;* 52, 367-373.

Wray J., and Radley-Smith, R. (2004). Depression in Pediatric Patients Before and 1 Year after Heart or Heart-Lung Transplantation. *J Heart Lung Transplant;* 23(9): 1103-10.

Wu, J.C., and Bunny, W.E. (1990). The Biological Basis of an Anti-depressant Response to Sleep Deprivation and Relapse: Review and Hypothesis. *American Journal of Psychiatry;* 147, 14-21.

Yapko, Michael, D. (1997). The Art of Avoiding Depression, Published by Psychology Today: May/June, 1997.

Zimmerman, M., Coryell, W., Stangl, D., and Phohl, B. (1987). Validity of an Operational Definition for Neurotoic Unipolar Major Depression. *Journal of Affective Disorders;* 12, 29-40.

Index